D0628171

Put Your Health
in Your Own Hands

Put Your Health in Your Own Hands

Natural Solutions
that Create Amazing Health

To Mick

Be Well

Bob

Bob Huttinga, PA-C, CNHP

First edition copyright © 2014 Bob Huttinga

All rights reserved. No part of this publication may be reproduced, stored in a retrieval system, or transmitted in any form or by any means, electronic, mechanical, photocopying, recording, or otherwise, without the prior written permission of the publisher.

ISBN: 978-0-578-13984-5

The Healing Center of Lakeview
332 S. Lincoln Ave.
Lakeview, Michigan 48850
(989) 352-6500 (O) (989) 352-6273 (F)
www.thehealingcenteroflakeview.com
bobhuttinga@healingcenter.biz

Printed in the United States of America

Dedication

I dedicate this book to my wife, Barbara Kay. She has been the wind beneath my wings for over 10 years. She is not only my loving spouse but also my business partner. It was she who gave me the title for the newspaper column and the book. She has been my inspiration and an occasional kick in the seat of the pants to do the things that must be done. Without her, this project would never have been published.

Secondary dedication is to my readers… to all of you who are searching, hoping to find an answer to those many questions you have about your life and your health. May this book start you on the path or help you continue your travels to find that answer.

Remember life is a journey.

This book is not the final destination. It is a depot, a port, an airport. It will help you find the next station, the next stop, the next point of interest.

Be well and Put Your Health in Your Own Hands!

Contents

Acknowledgements

THIS is my chance to thank all those who helped me write this book. The idea started after I had been writing a newspaper column for the local newspaper, *Lakeview Area News*. So I give thanks to editor Linda Hutchins for giving me space in the paper to write my views and experiences on the topic of natural health.

Thanks to my parents, Alko and Alice Huttinga, for great parenting, strong morals and values, a Christian background, as well as a focus on college and higher education. Their strong work ethic has been both a strength and a weakness. One of their sayings still rings in my ears, "God helps those who help themselves." That concept has been a driving force in the success of my life, but that also became the basis for my negative "workaholic" traits.

Many thanks to my proofreaders and local editors: Eunice Norwood, Megan Stevens, Anne Wakenhut, Sheral Simon, and Bonnie Knopf Cour. My thanks to the Chariti Withey for the front cover photograph. I am grateful for a great focus group who read this book and gave me much insight into how to clearly say what I wanted to say. Special thanks go to Robert Weir who did the final editing and mentored me through the publishing process.

My medical training was influenced by many people. The physicians from Lakeview Medical Center (1976–1981), Drs. Bruce Bennett, Richard Yerian, Caesar Bonet, John London, and Robert Painter, helped shape the basic platform upon which I practice my version of health care. Later, Drs. Grant and Tammy Born of the Born Clinic in Grand Rapids, Michigan, planted, watered, and fertilized the seeds of natural health and were a big influence on my thinking. Dr. Jackie Featherly, ND, (Let's Get Healthy, Edmore, Michigan) and Dr. Bessheen Baker, ND, (NITE Institute, Mount Pleasant, Michigan) were instrumental in my understanding of herbs and homeopathy. Dr. Robin Murphy, ND, (Lotus Institute, Blacksburg, Virginia) provided the foundation for my knowledge of homeopathy. Dr. Samuel Hahnemann

(1755–1843), who created the art of homeopathy, definitely needs to take a bow for his work two centuries ago.

My mental, emotional, and spiritual development has had many assists along the way. A few years ago when we moved from one home to another, I found I had 27 feet of books on shelves that I had read over the years. I am sure there are many more that were loaned out or left behind for someone else's growth. A few of the greats are Wayne Dyer, Jose Silva, Dale Carnegie, Neville Goddard, and Napoleon Hill. These authors have had a huge influence on my thinking and understanding of people and the world in which we live.

Thanks to God and the many unseen hands in the spiritual world for the gentle intuitions and the occasional whacks on the side of the head that have brought me to this point in my life.

Author's Note

PUT *Your Health in Your Own Hands* started as a newspaper column, written over a five-year period according to topics that seemed most relevant at the time. For this book, I've taken them out of chronological order and reorganized them into a few logical groups. Because of the origin of the material, there is some repetition of important material to imprint it more powerfully in your brain. Therefore, this is not just another nice, fluffy book but valuable information you can use to *put your health in your own hands*. For easier reference, helpful terms are alphabetically indexed in the back of the book.

This is my first book. There have been times when I think it will also be my last. But, in reality, I know that is not true. I have acquired a huge amount of training and understanding about human nature, why we are here, and how to remain healthy in body, mind, and spirit. More books are already forming in my mind.

It should be noted that very little of this book is based on proven research. It is my own observation, study, and intuition over 40 years of reading many books and working with thousands of patients in many different clinical settings.

We are in an information age. People want to be more informed and are beginning to take more responsibility for their own health and wellness. They just need to know what to do. They also want trustworthy information. I will continue to pass on important, easy-to-understand guidelines about personal health in this crazy world.

To my colleagues in the medical field

WE have been blessed with great knowledge. Most of us entered the field of the healing arts with some altruistic ideal that we could make a difference in the lives of our patients. Most of us do that to varying degrees every day. Unfortunately, I found as I grew older that I became more jaded by the system, by insurance companies, and by patients themselves. I found that I was getting caught up in treating numbers, not patients. I became more focused on the business of medicine instead of the healing aspects of health care.

Natural medicine has been a great gift to me. With it, I can return to that ideal. I also have many more tools to use for those functional conditions that drive most health care providers crazy. In traditional medicine, we need a diagnosis that is evidence-base. However, we constantly encounter many people who have complaints and symptoms with no evidence based findings.

Not knowing what to do with these people is a huge source of frustration for patients and providers alike. One solution is to look at tools such as herbs, homeopathy, and hypnosis, which are often effective for those functional conditions with no pathological findings. Another important need is more patient education so people can put *their* health into *their* own hands. We, in the medical field, must function as coaches and educators.

Disclaimer

IN the pages of this book are many recommendations. To the best of my knowledge, the things that I have written about are safe, time-tested suggestions. But they are only suggestions. It is up to you to put your health in your own hands. You are responsible. You are the performer, the star, the actor in your own life. It is up to you to take these suggestions and use them with common sense. I am your coach. If something I say does not make sense to you, then disregard it, or research it, or discuss it with a professional who is qualified in that area. Only use these suggestions if they resonate with your own thinking. Put *your* health in *your* own hands.

Where are we going?

BECAUSE it helps to know where we are going before we begin a journey, here is the summary of our trip and our destination.

Putting your heath in your own hands is the holistic concept we must embrace as our world shifts in consciousness. We, as human beings, have many parts that we call *self*: physical, mental, emotional, spiritual, parent, child, employee, business owner, female, male, etc.

There is a seagoing, military term, *muster*, which means "to gather." We need to gather ourselves together; to get all of our parts flying in formation. To get our "*selfs*" together, we must learn to muster our parts.

To become responsible for our own selves, we *must* learn to:

- Cleanse our bodies of toxins
- Stop adding to the toxic load
- Rebuild damaged tissues
- Control our minds
- Focus and concentrate
- Slow down and relax
- Enhance our memories
- Use our negative emotions to focus on what we really, really want
- Feel good all the time
- Connect with our spirit and with the spirit of our Higher Power

This book is a tool, a starting place, an introduction.
My purpose is:

- To introduce you to the possibilities that will help you step out of your current comfort zone of old, detrimental thoughts and actions that interfere with your health

- To help you understand that there are many ways to maintain your health
- To give you one more little nudge toward self-awareness and understanding that you have unlimited potential for perfect health
- To help you know that you can be, do, and have anything you desire to be, do, or have

All you need to do is put your health—physical, mental, emotional, and spiritual—in your own hands and then *muster* all your parts into an integrated whole. Hopefully, this book will prove to be a guide, a focusing tool, and an ongoing reference as you find your way to wholeness.

Introduction

A few years ago, I had the good fortune to meet a man who was 103 years old. He drove himself to the Gratiot Medical Center Urgent Care Clinic because he had cut his finger working in his workshop. He was taking no medicine and was mentally very sharp. While I was working to repair his finger, I asked him, "What is your secret to your long and healthy life?" His reply was very enlightening. "I stayed away from you darn doctors!" We had a good laugh about that.

This story is not meant to put down doctors, but it illustrates that there are many alternatives. Healthy people over 80 years of age have their own opinions as to why they have reached that age in good health. Two things are almost always present: they are usually non-smokers, and they have a busy, active lifestyle. The purpose of this book is to explore things we can do, no matter what our age, to increase not only the length but the quality of our lives.

The famous philosopher Socrates once said, "It is the nature of an entity that determines what it will do and what it can do." This means, if one human being can do something, then any other human being can learn to do that also. So if one person can live to be over 103 years of age, in perfect health, then anyone else can learn to do that too.

Put your health in your own hands

I was raised in a small farm community near Bozeman, Montana. Life was fairly simple. Dad worked at the local grain elevator and farmed on the side. Mom ran the household and raised four kids. Starting at an early age, my brothers and I helped a lot with the farm, cutting firewood, doing chores and field work.

Mom struggled with her weight her whole life, as did her mother. Dad's family was generally tall and thin. Because of her weight concerns, Mom

3

became very health conscious and did the best she could to feed us organic, home-grown food.

My parents were poorly educated, but their focus was that we were going to get an education, and there was never a doubt that I would go to college. So at age 17, I moved to Grand Rapids, Michigan, to attend Calvin College. There, I studied biology and chemistry, taking pre-med classes. But due to past programming, I had very poor self-esteem and could never really see myself as a doctor. I decided to study botany at Calvin College, then return to Montana, and go into forestry.

Yet I was destined for a different path. I had to work full time to pay for school and I got a job as an orderly working in a nursing home. I worked third shift and found that I loved working with these older people. Feeding them, bathing them, and cleaning up the poopy messes did not bother me at all. This job renewed my interest in health care. After a year, I moved up to a job in the hospital, again as an orderly and later as an on-the-job trained respiratory therapist. I really liked that work, doing not only patient care but helping in the emergency room. There, I met a young resident physician who had been in the military. He introduced me to the idea of becoming a physician assistant (PA). The Army and Air Force had started training corpsmen, mostly from Vietnam, to go on to work with doctors, but the concept of being a PA wasn't known in civilian life.

So, in 1974, I applied to the program at Western Michigan University in Kalamazoo, Michigan, and was accepted into a class of 22 students, the school's second physician assistant class. I worked full time at the hospital as a respiratory therapist, studied like a mad man, and took my grade point average from average to exceptional.

The program was very new, so we had to find our own family practice internship. Because my wife's family was from Grand Rapids, just an hour north of Kalamazoo, I wanted to live in that general area. I sent letters to 50 doctors and small hospitals within 50 miles. I only received one letter back. Why? No one knew what a PA was! There was not even any legislation or a governing body to organize and create standards for the profession.

That one doctor who replied was Dr. Richard Yerian, DO. He also had been in the military and knew about PAs. He worked with a group of four other physicians, Drs. Bennett, London, Bonet, and Painter, in Lakeview, a small rural community an hour north of Grand Rapids at the edge of that 50 mile radius I had targeted.

These doctors invited me and my wife, who was five months pregnant, for an interview and accepted me to spend four months with them in a family practice internship. By the end of that time, they offered me a job. I was in heaven.

The next five years were a fabulous learning and working experience. We did surgeries in the mornings in a small local hospital and saw patients in the afternoons in the clinic. These men were true healers as well as good technicians.

It was during this time that I began to notice the body-mind connection. I also noticed much depression in the community. We had very poor medicines for mental health conditions and I did a lot of counseling. People usually felt better just talking things over, and I gained the perception that doctors' lack of awareness regarding the connection between body and mind was a huge weakness in the medical system.

We wanted our children educated in Christian schools. So after five years at Lakeview Medical Center, we moved to Grand Rapids where I took a job with General Motors (GM), working in occupational health at one of the local GM plants. That was great work. I helped develop an ergonomics program and worked with engineers to modify jobs to reduce injuries. Although I really liked the work, it was also very political and very stressful. I began to drink alcohol as self-medication because no one had ever taught me how to relax. I never knew that I could do something about stress besides taking a pill or alcohol. During this time, I took a four-hour stress management class that truly changed my life.

Within a few weeks of practicing these relaxation techniques, I was able to normalize my blood pressure, heal an ulcer, and stop medicating myself in a destructive manner. I found this so beneficial that I went on to study and later teach The Silva Method of Mind Development and Stress Control, a program that teaches advanced relaxation, meditation, and mental/emotional problem solving. I highly recommend this method to anyone trying to deal with and manage stress in their lives.

Unfortunately, my first marriage ended after 19 years. After being single a few years, I remarried. Going way off my path of destiny, I spent ten years drinking, partying, and generally having a "good" time. A second divorce, which was a great whack on the side of the head, brought me back on track.

I believe that, before we are born, our soul creates a destiny that I call our "birth vision." This is an outline for our life and what we plan to accomplish. But, sometimes, we become like rudderless ships forgetting our objective and our birth vision. Then, because this is a map or plan we must follow, we get redirected by our higher power.

In early 2003, I became reacquainted with Barb. We had met a couple years before, when she had done three emotional release massages on me during the pain of the second divorce. These had been very successful to help me eliminate the effects of grief and loss.

Later that year, we married. We actually got married twice, once locally and a second time in Egypt in the king's chamber of the Great Pyramid of Giza. Barb was working as a massage therapist, her second career after toxicity from 35 years of styling hair had made her very ill. By the time we married, she had recovered and was doing very well.

One night, I asked her, "What do you want to do with the rest of your life?" She said, "I want to open a healing center." That statement impregnated an idea that eventually hatched to become The Healing Center in Lakeview, Michigan, just a few blocks from where I started my medical work nearly 30 years earlier. Yes, I felt like I was back on track.

We found a 110-year-old building and totally renovated it, creating a holistic healing place where we offer traditional medicine, naturopathic medicine (essential oils and herbs), energy medicine, homeopathy, hypnosis, metaphysical healing, and much more.

After two years of hard work renovating the building, we opened and began the task of marketing ourselves. As with any new venture, we had a few struggles, but this helped us hone our vision of what we really wanted. One day, I suggested to Barb that we needed a slogan for The Healing Center. After incubating ideas for a while, she came up with "Put Your Health in Your Own Hands."

Putting your health in your own hands is also a general trend in natural health care. People today are much more aware of what is going on with their own bodies and want some control of their health and their health care.

Some people still want the doctor to make all the decisions, but more and more are saying, "No, I want to know why. I need to understand what this medicine does, why I need it, and what harm it can cause."

I agree with the intent behind these questions.

In natural health, the individual *must* be involved. He or she must be aware of all degrees of medical intervention from external and internal remedies to invasive surgeries.

At The Healing Center, we think nutrition should be the first line of treatment. Next, we use cleansing and building with vitamins, minerals, and herbs. Then, we have homeopathic remedies, Bach Flower remedies, and essential oils, which stimulate the body's own healing capability. Mental and emotional clearing and spiritual balance are vital. And, finally, we believe that prescription medicine and surgery should be used only for life-threatening illnesses and if there is too much tissue damage for natural methods to repair.

Throughout history, people have generally cared for themselves. But in the last 40 or 50 years, Western society has become too dependent on the doctor and high-tech medicine. I suggest that you ask your doctor, "Why do I need to be on all these medicines?" and "What are the side effects?" Pay attention to the answers.

If you are on prescription medicine, do not stop them without your doctor's knowledge. But you can make nutritional changes, cleanse and build your body with natural treatments. Then, as your laboratory test results get better, talk again with your doctor about how and when you can begin to wean off the medicines.

It is always best to do this with your doctor's supervision. It is sad, though, that some people are afraid to tell the doctor they want to do something different. I saw a new patient recently who wanted to go off Zocor, a common medication to lower cholesterol. His doctor agreed. His cholesterol went up to 230 with an LDL of 120. The doctor wanted him to restart the Zocor. Instead, the patient started an herbal treatment. The recheck numbers were very good (198, 104 respectively). But then he was afraid to tell the doctor what he was doing. Your doctor should be your coach. Find one who will be your guide, not a dictator. Being involved in your own health care improves both quality and length of life.

Of course, this isn't a philosophy that I would have imagined, much less adopted, while a young man in Montana, in college, or even early in my medical career. But it is a philosophy by which I live my life today and encourage others to do the same. After some very interesting detours and distractions, I have reconnected with my birth vision.

What is your path?

Each of our lives is a path with many twists and turns. The decisions we make as we go along the road determine what our futures will look like. It is fun to look back and see how certain choices brought us to the place we are today.

Later on, we will ask you to examine your life's path and create a timeline of emotional and physical trauma you have encountered. This will help you to fix the current effects of some of those events from the past.

Constitutional Health:
What you were born with

WE are born with a certain level of health, based on our genetics and the effects of our mother's pregnancy. This starting point is called *constitutional health*. There are many things we can do to maintain this level of health so we will have a long and fruitful life.

What is health?

Traditional Western medicine would say that good health is the absence of disease. But being healthy really is having adequate vital energy every day to do the things you want to do with no limitations.

Even before birth, we begin to be touched by the world around us. There is evidence that a human fetus "hears" at four months. So, pregnant moms, remember to keep your environment clean and peaceful. And, dads, be respectful, quiet, and courteous to both the woman with whom you are creating this child and the baby within her.

After birth, toxic exposures, infections, physical trauma, surgery, and emotional shocks all begin to exert their influence on our constitution. We either recover fully or we only partially recover from the effects of these external factors.

As we go through the years, these constant impacts create a gradual reduction in our level of health. If our recovery and self-healing potentials are greater than the insults to our body, mind, and spirit, then we will retain a reasonably good level of health. If the insults (often self-inflicted) are greater than our self-healing ability, we will begin to experience acute and then chronic illness, which could eventually become degenerative beyond the point of repair. These conditions are then named as diseases (in modern holistic language "dis-ease" or the "absence of ease") and become known as pathological conditions.

As parents, we do our best to maintain a good fetal environment for our child. Then, as the child grows from infancy to adulthood, we do our best to reduce toxins, provide good water, food, and so on. Sometimes we can reduce physical and emotional shocks. We encourage the growing child to avoid tobacco, alcohol, caffeine, sweets, and things that are known to be detrimental.

Caring for ourselves as parents, we can do periodic cleanses to remove accumulated toxins. We can use prayer and meditation to remove the emotional shocks affecting our mind and spirit. By finding the correct homeopathic medicine and Bach Flower remedy, we can remove the bad effects of physical and emotional trauma. Foods, herbs, and natural methods are our best method of building the self-healing and recovery mechanisms that reside within us.

So, as we progress through our lives, things happen to us. Physical and emotional traumas happen that reduce our level of health. If we totally recover to our constitutional level of health, that is great. But often we do not totally recover to the same level we were before the event, and, gradually, as more events occur, we see continuing reduction in our over-all level of health.

In addition to this ongoing reduction in our level of health, we might also engage in activities and habits that become obstacles to our recovery. These are things we do physically, mentally, emotionally, and spiritually that keep us stuck in illness and disease. Natural health is about removing those *obstacles to recovery* so the body and mind can return to its previously healthy state, which it knows how to do very well. We just need to get out of the way.

Finally, we could get to a point where tissue damage begins to occur during an event. This physical damage is called pathology and it refers to diseases and diagnoses. Natural treatments can assist to some degree to reverse the damage or make it easier to live with these aches and pains. Our mission is to find the answer *before* the pathology occurs and to build or cleanse the body back to its naturally healthy state.

Body-Mind-Spirit connection

When I started in medicine 38 years ago in physician assistant (PA) school, I learned mostly about the physical body and its problems. We studied a little psychology but very little about how the mind works and nothing about the body-mind-spirit connection.

I noticed that many physical illnesses were caused by stress and how we think. Over the years, I began to understand that our mind is the connecting link between our body and our spiritual self. When we learn how to control our thoughts, our bodies become more whole because we are more connected to our spiritual side.

Many of us have religious beliefs that we think as human beings help us develop our spiritual side. But let's suppose it is the opposite: maybe we are spiritual beings trying to become more human. If that is the case, then it is extremely important to learn how our mind works. When we have that understanding, our spiritual part, which knows how to be perfect, can connect with our bodies. It can then instruct our bodies on ways to become healthy and happy every day that we are alive.

We are very capable of learning to consciously control our thoughts. We can then focus on solutions instead of problems, on desirable outcomes instead of the worst case scenarios, and on the good in people instead of their faults.

As we begin to listen to the still small voice of intuition that is constantly guiding us, we discover that intuition comes as mental pictures, self-talk, or feelings. This is the perfect inner spiritual part of us trying to guide our bodies to do the correct thing for the best outcome for all concerned.

It is important to learn as much as possible about our complete selves, about our entire body-mind-spirit connection.

How can we do this? Read books, listen to tapes, or attend classes. Listen to your intuition; it is guiding you. Go to a bookstore and just cruise through the self-help or natural health section; some book that you need will just jump off the shelf into your hands. Read that and begin to understand that, in order to be healthy, we need to look at our whole being.

Also, as you read this book, you will find that, in the course of these pages, I will explain the basics of homeopathy and how it works. Then some of these early references to homeopathic remedies will make more sense.

The cycles of life

If you can say, "I have never been well since I hit my head on that beam," then you have found the underlying cause of the symptoms. We call this the "etiology of your illness." Once you find the origin of your current symptoms, then you will want to find a solution that will correct that situation.

A way to gain an understanding of the origin of your symptoms is to construct a timeline of all emotional, infectious, accidental, surgical, and physical events from conception until now that still affect your life.

Every living thing has a natural life cycle during which it is born, grows to maturity, then gradually deteriorates, and eventually dies. During our youth and the early adult years, we experience anabolic (build up) cycles during which our body is continuously building and getting stronger. Then, in our later decades, we have catabolic (break down) cycles that deteriorate and weaken the body.

There are a multitude of ideas about this, and every author and researcher on this subject has his or her own ideas about how long these cycles last and how often they repeat. The concept that most fits my understanding is borrowed from Jose Silva, the founder of The Silva Method of Mind Development and Stress Control.

Silva believed that, on average, we go through seven-year cycles. During that time, all of our tissues turn over so we have a completely new body. Some cells, such as the red blood cells, have shorter cycles and change every few days. Some, like nerve cells, have longer cycles and turn over every seven years.

Silva felt that, from birth to age 49, we go through a series of seven anabolic cycles followed by another series of seven catabolic cycles for a total potential life span of 98 years.

The rest of this section defines some of the characteristics of each phase in the cycles of life. Please read it carefully, then stop reading and construct a timeline of your life. I believe you will find that doing this exercise will help you determine the cause of many of your current health issues.

Prenatal

To ensure that you have a healthy baby, there are some important things to know before you get pregnant and during the pregnancy. Six months prior to getting pregnant, both parents should be doing some things to prepare. (According to Weston A. Price, in primitive cultures, parents would prepare for two years.) Supplements high in natural vitamin B from alfalfa and docosahexaenoic acid (DHA) from omega-3 fish oil are crucial for normal brain development in the fetus.

Avoidance of caffeine, alcohol, tobacco, and soda pop are very important because these dehydrate the system. When the body of the pregnant mom becomes chronically dehydrated, she begins to develop adrenal fatigue. At the third trimester, the fetal adrenal glands start working to the point where they begin to supply adrenal hormones to the mom. She begins to feel really good for the remainder of the pregnancy. After the baby is born, the mother again begins to experience adrenal fatigue, which causes depression, fatigue, and irritability. The baby, meanwhile, is over-producing adrenaline for its little body size and begins having sleep issues as well as heart and gastro-intestinal problems. All of this will readjust over time. But remember, adequate hydration and avoidance of carbonated and caffeinated beverages will help to avoid this issue.

In his book, *The Power of Sound*, Joshua Leeds gives remarkable information on how sound and the things we say around the pregnant mom influence the baby after the fourth month. Exposure to classical music has been shown to enhance brain development and actually will later improve the child's ability to perform math and logical reasoning.

Case Study: AB was a 20-month-old boy who was brought to my office with severe separation anxiety, night terrors, and difficulty sleeping. When his mother was six months pregnant, AB's father abandoned them for two weeks, leaving his mother stranded and afraid. Homeopathic Pulsatilla is the remedy that the mother should have had to relieve her feelings of abandonment and fear during the pregnancy. If she had taken the Pulsatilla when this happened, AB would have been a happier baby.

I gave AB a few doses of homeopathic Pulsatilla. That resolved that situation permanently. There are several other remedies that could have been used, but I chose this remedy based on the "provings" or experiences of many homeopathic practitioners before me.

Author's Note: Most homeopathic remedies can be taken during pregnancy, however consult a professional before taking any medication during pregnancy.

In the early 1980s, Joseph and Jitsuko Susedik demonstrated that educating their yet-to-be-born children was not only possible but reproducible. Throughout the whole pregnancy, both parents "talked" to their baby, explaining everything they were doing throughout their daily routines. In the last three or four months, the mother assigned a subject to each day of the week. Monday was geography day, Tuesday was math day, Wednesday was history day, and so forth. Each day of the week, she taught the baby some "lesson" by going to a museum or reading a book on that subject. After, birth the child recognized information as familiar rather than brand new and unfamiliar. This organized prenatal teaching program resulted in highly gifted children.

Good nutrition, natural vitamins, omega-3 fish oil, adequate sunshine, the right amount of water, and exercise are all very important for the development of a healthy baby. A little planning and a few changes can dramatically improve the developing mental and physical health of your baby and greatly reduce the chances for birth defects and other health risks.

Birth to 7 Years

In this age range, huge amounts of learning takes place. The child's brain produces large amounts of alpha brain waves that cause the child to be open and receptive to everything around them. The child is much like someone under hypnosis and absorbs everything. During this stage, the child is almost totally dependent on someone else for his or her survival.

If there are problems in this cycle and if no cause can be found for the issues, the mother should review the history of the pregnancy. If there were events during the pregnancy, labor, or delivery that might be the source, then the infant or toddler should be given the same homeopathic remedy that the mother needed during that time.

Case Study: DB was a 6-year-old brought to The Healing Center by his mother, who is a grade school principal. DB had severe separation anxiety, which had not subsided as he experienced more and more time away from his parents. In all other aspects, he was normal, but he would cry and scream and throw a full-blown tantrum for two to three hours whenever his mother would leave him. School was an ordeal. Mom would deliver him to school and the teacher would have to carry him, kicking and screaming, to the classroom.

A careful history revealed that, during delivery, the mother had had a nearly fatal allergic reaction to a narcotic pain medication. As a result, I surmised that the infant also had a near-death experience. This programmed his body to produce fight-or-flight chemicals to deal with that emotional trauma. He continued to trigger the fight-or-flight reaction any time he felt separation from his life source.

Because of his mother's reaction to the narcotic, I gave him a homeopathic remedy that we use for narcotic withdrawal. A single dose of this medication removed all the anxiety associated with his mother leaving him. The morning after the remedy was given, his mother drove him to school. When they arrived at his school, he jumped out of the car, waving and saying, "Bye, Mom. I love you." Then he reached back into the car and, patting her hand, said, "You will be alright." The mom, of course, was astounded, ecstatic, and actually felt a little loss for a short time because he had been so connected to her prior to that moment. But she recovered from that very quickly.

This dramatic recovery and response to a single dose of homeopathy is rare. More often, the changes are gradual with steady improvement over time. I was amazed myself to see the power of this treatment. I am reminded of Dr. Bennett's advice to me many years ago, "all the answers are in the patient's story."

8 to 14 Years

During these years, the child begins to produce more beta brain waves and fewer alpha brain waves, becoming more discerning and judgmental. This cycle is a preparation stage for adult decision making. Children usually become more independent and learn to make right choices. If there are health or behavior problems, it is often because the child is stuck in previous emotional or physical trauma that was imprinted in the past.

Case Study: HS was a teenager with learning and behavior issues and an inability to focus. These were new and had been going on for just a few weeks, but already his grades were slipping. The family doctor had suggested medications for attention deficit disorder (ADD). His mother disagreed and came seeking a natural remedy. A careful study of the boy's recent history revealed that, a few weeks before, he had been hit hard in the head while playing football. Homeopathic Natrum Sulphuricum 30C, given under the tongue twice a day for about a week, totally resolved the learning and behavioral issues.

Events such as having your "bell rung" are cumulative and, if not cleared, can influence the rest of our lives.

15 to 21 Years

This is the transition stage when a young person grows to adult survival and being independent of parents and others. It is at this time when life-long patterns, based on prior experience, begin to emerge. If things are not going well, they can be changed with nutritional changes, homeopathic remedies, essential oils, natural healing, meditation, and mental reprogramming.

Food allergies and ingestion of toxins, including antibiotics and steroids that are often given to children, might also be a factor in the health of a young adult.

Case Study: JH is one of my teenage patients. He has multiple food sensitivities. One of the worst is high fructose corn syrup. The following is an edited version of an article from a newsletter written by Dr. Bessheen Baker, ND, of Naturopathic Institute of Therapies & Education in Mount Pleasant, Michigan. It is an account of this young man's journey over the past ten years.

When JH was in the first grade, he started to act differently. Instead of being the very loving, sweet and gentle spirit that he normally was, he started having what his mom referred to as "meltdowns," during which he would come home from school and be very mean and angry.

At first, his parents thought he was having problems with his teacher, but that didn't seem to be the issue. The meltdowns worsened. He would lash out, having violent rages, punching walls, shaking his bed, tearing things apart, hitting his parents, and threatening to kill them. His mom had bruises from these rages. On the worst days, his dad stayed home from his work and restrained him.

These poor parents wondered what they were doing wrong. And the sweet little boy would sob after the rage was over. He would apologize, saying he couldn't help it, that something came over him. He also wondered what was wrong. The situation got so bad that the parents, who had two other children, questioned whether it was safe for him to continue to stay in the home and if they should send him away.

One of the last episodes occurred after the mom had bought some chocolate corn puff cereal for a treat and the boy, by then a teenager, had eaten quite a lot. When one of the worst rages followed, the mom called her naturopath, Dr. Bessheen Baker, ND, and asked if there was anything natural that could help this problem.

Dr. Baker said to immediately avoid all high fructose corn syrup and corn products. What happened next was a miracle. An amazing turnaround occurred, and the good-natured boy returned. He still has normal teenage behavior, but there are no violent rages. Mom can tell when he's had a food with corn syrup in it. The boy reads labels now and avoids things that have corn syrup listed in the ingredients.

That little boy is now a teenager and has been able to be himself for the past few years. In looking back, the family realized that, in first grade, he started eating school lunches that contained high fructose corn syrup.

This is truly an eye opening account of how seriously corn syrup, or any chemical additive, could impact the health of one person, not to mention the effect it has on an entire family. It is also an inspiring story of how we can choose to take responsibility for our own health and heal ourselves on all levels, putting our health into our own hands.

22 to 49 Years

This is the life stage of raising children and making careers, a time when the effects of earlier life stages become impactful and visible in a positive or a negative way.

Fatherly Advice: When I was in my early 20s, I called my father to ask if I could borrow $2,000 for a down payment on a lake lot in northern Michigan. His very quick answer was, "I have the money, but I am not going to loan it to you." "Why not?" I asked. He said, "Two reasons: First, you are very capable of raising this money yourself. If you really want it and the deal is right, you will find a way. Second, if I do this, then every time you need money, you will think I am the bank. I am not your bank. You are very capable to find a way to do this yourself."

At first, I was angry. Then I realized what he had done. He had given me his blessing and told me I was capable. Not once, but twice. He thought I had what it took to care for myself. Wow. He also gave me a great lesson that I have used with my children. I was creating my life. Why would he want to take away an opportunity for me to learn a great lesson and feel the empowerment of accomplishment.

The voice of my father saying, "You can do it," has rung in my ears thousands of times in my life. Often when I wanted to give up and quit, I heard his words. This is the stage of life in which most people have their greatest successes, either in raising a family or career and business.

50 to 98 Years

Even though age 50 is the beginning of the catabolic (break-down) cycles, this is the time when people are often at the height of their careers and are still looking forward to many great ventures in the fifth, sixth, seventh, and even eighth decade. This is also a time when many people begin to feel the aches and pains of life's effects from earlier years. I remember what my old mentor Dr. Bruce Bennett used to say, "It is not your age; it is just your mileage."

Before running to the doctor for prescription medications, read on in this book and learn about many natural remedies to:

- Change what you eat for better health.
- Utilize cleanses to remove toxins.
- Add vitamin and herbal supplements to build your body.

- Use essential oils and homeopathic medicines to treat the symptoms.
- Take control of your health.

If all that fails, you could need pharmaceutical medicine prescribed by a medical doctor. But remember that prescription medicines are designed to force the body to try to do something different than it wants to do. These side effects generally do not occur when a person implements changes using nutrition, supplements, herbs, essential oils, or homeopathy.

The timeline of health

Now, I would like you to do something. This book is about getting results, putting your health in your own hands. So get some paper and a pen and begin to construct your timeline of major events that might have affected your health.

Include physical trauma, accidents, injuries, surgeries, serious infections, and allergic reactions.

Also include emotional traumas: grief, broken attachments, real or imagined lost love, abandonment or feeling forsaken or helpless, mortification, humiliation, embarrassment, guilt, being teased excessively, rape, abuse, fright, bad news, worry or anticipation of bad things happening, disappointment, burnout or over-exertion of the mind, expressed or suppressed anger, homesickness, jealousy, being dishonest or lack of integrity by others.

Later in this book, we will address how to correct the latent effects of these events. Ideas in the text will likely jog your memory, so continue to fill in the timeline as you read.

Evolution

When I was growing up, we believed in creation, so when we hear the word "evolution," we put our guard up, thinking that this concept was evil. In fact, many religions hold that idea. But evolution simply means change. And that is something we all must do.

When we are born, we are basically animals and our whole purpose is to survive, both personally and as a species. We have animalistic survival instincts programmed into our DNA. So we compete and fight (cry, scream, and throw tantrums when a child) in order to ensure that we get what we need. We also express our innate cuteness in order to gain cuddling and touch.

As we grow up, we emerge into a more humanistic state. We begin to use the morals and values we learned from our parents, teachers, churches, and society. Most of us get to a point when we know that we and the species will survive and we begin to focus on the human characteristics of love, compassion, cooperation, and the good of all concerned.

The next phase of change is an awareness of our spiritual part. Sometime between childhood and death, most of us become aware of a divine, higher power within. We reach that point in many ways. For some, it is part of religious training as children. For others, it might be a near-death experience. Maybe it is the Twelve-Step program of Alcoholics Anonymous. Perhaps the diagnosis of a terminal illness brings us to spiritual awareness. There are countless experiences of awakening to our spirituality.

In the animal and human states, we are often not aware of this divine part of us. If we are aware, we feel that this higher power is outside of us. As we evolve and grow in our spiritual awareness, we realize that this inner divine power is a vital force that actually powers our system. Sure, the organs and tissues all play their role in the physical form but, without this divine spark, often called the soul, we could not and would not exist.

In holistic medicine, we pay attention to this spiritual part because it has such a huge impact on the physical and mental. In homeopathy, we believe that this vital spiritual energy produces the symptoms that guide us to the correct remedy to bring the complete being—our body, mind, and spirit—back into alignment and wholeness.

So realize that we are evolving beings from animal to human to spirit. Our state shifts with the events in our lives. We can be God-like one minute and a homicidal animal the next. My goal is to see people move more in the direction of being highly evolved spiritual beings, leaving behind the old animalist ways, which are based on old programming. Our physical, mental, and spiritual health are inseparable.

Indigo Children

In 1992, a book titled *Indigo Children* was written by Lee Carroll and Jan Taber who had observed a very interesting thing in some children. A person they worked with had a condition known as synesthesia. Synesthesia is a sensation produced in one physical sense when a stimulus is applied to another physical sense, such as when the hearing of a certain sound induces the visualization of a certain color. This person saw the color indigo around these children when she heard them speak. Hence, the title of the book and the name "Indigos" that is given to these children.

This indigo color is the electromagnetic field or aura that surrounds all of us, a subject that I will explain later in great detail. These children were unusually intelligent and mature. Some know things before they happen.

The following two case studies might seem a bit far-fetched, but remain open minded as much as possible. Like my mentor, Jose Silva, used to say, "Could be…." as he advised that we just reserve judgment until we have more information.

Case Study: One indigo child I know calls her great-grandmother "Kitty." This was a pet name the elder woman's father used for her when she was a child. No one had called her that for over 50 years and the child had never met the great-grandfather.

Case Study: I have a patient, CM, who, by the age of five, knew a great deal of accurate information about Europe. He knew the names of counties and roads even though he could not read and had never been there. His mother took him to a medium, who said he had been a WWI soldier stationed in Europe in a former life.

Carroll and Tabor describe children in China who have telekinesis, the ability to move objects with their minds. They also talk about other children who can hold a book to their head and know its content, without reading it. Some of these kids see and talk to angels and spirits.

Most indigo children have an unusual connection to nature and are almost overly concerned about the environment. All seem to be very connected to animals. Some are wizards with machines and electronics. Many are diagnosed with attention deficit disorder (ADD) and autism. Some have major behavior problems.

We do not know exactly what the presence of indigos in our world means for the advancement of civilization or evolution of the human species, but

Carroll and Tabor feel that these changes are happening to help the new generations handle the huge amounts of information and technology that are soon to be invented.

It is important to understand these indigo children are different but not defective. Sometimes, they need different types of education than presently found in our standard educational systems. Often, they respond to negotiation rather than discipline and to natural remedies better than to prescription medications. For more information, read Carroll and Taber's book, *Indigo Children.*

Events that Reduce Our Level of Health

A S we go through life there are cycles, ups and downs, illnesses, traumas (physical and emotional), surgeries, allergies, and circumstances that reduce our constitutional health. Our goal is to totally recover after each of these events and return to our ideal health.

If there is nothing wrong, why do I feel so bad?

This is a question I have heard many times in my nearly 40 years as a physician assistant. The answer lies in the study of how illnesses progress and how traditional medicine defines illness.

In general, we could name three stages of health:

First stage: *healthy and well* means having enough vital energy every day to do the things we desire to do with no limitations. This is the stage of health we all want to be in.

Second stage: *functional condition* is limbo-land in which we feel bad, have a lot of symptoms, but yet nothing shows up on medical tests. Many people find themselves in this stage.

Third stage: *pathological conditions* mean that diseases and illnesses have been recognized by observation of damaged tissue and abnormal results on lab tests and x-rays. Because these illnesses have names, have been studied, and have evidence-based diagnoses, practitioners of traditional medicine can deal with them.

Remember: "It is not your age; it is just your mileage." Each time we have an acute illness, an injury, or an emotional shock and do not totally recover from those insults, we experience a reduction in our overall level of health. As a result, we start to see signs of stress on our genetically weakest systems. Long before actual tissue damage occurs, we enter this area of functional condition.

This functional stage is the condition in which nutrition, homeopathy, and natural health are most beneficial. Eating good food, avoiding the toxic additives, drinking adequate water, getting daily exercise, getting a massage, using herbs to cleanse and build, and taking supplements will help us return to the stage of being healthy and well.

> **Case Study:** KJ, age 35, felt ill for 18 months. Beginning two weeks after having had a flu shot, her symptoms of fatigue, joint stiffness, and muscle aches were sometimes debilitating to the point that she was often bed-bound. Recognizing that her symptoms were caused by her overactive immune system, which thought she had the flu rather than just controlled exposure to the flu virus, we treated her with a homeopathic Gelsemium 200C, a natural treatment for influenza, twice a day for five days. She fully recovered within a few weeks.

We need to learn to read the signs. The little aches and pain, the heartburn, the blurry vision, the occasional headache, the urinary troubles, the PMS are all signals from your body that changes need to be made. These symptoms are not diseases. They are simple signals. Learn to stop, look, and listen. Pay attention to what your body is telling you. Learn to fix the functional conditions before they become pathological problems that require prescription medicine and surgery.

Symptoms: What is your body telling you?

A symptom is a message from within our body. Much like the red light on the dashboard of our car that flashes "oil," a symptom increases our awareness that something needs correction.

In natural medicine, we know that the symptom also tells us what nutritional change, herb, essential oil, or homeopathic remedy can be used to correct the internal problem so the symptom will go away. When we get a pain, we should ask, "What is this symptom trying to tell me?"

- Heartburn usually means: "Do not eat that food." Or perhaps: "Do not eat so much of that food. Reduce the size of that big gut." Or, emotionally, "What is eating at me?"
- Constipation means: "Eat differently." "Drink more water." "Eat more foods that are high in fiber." It could be asking, "What am I emotionally holding on to?" or "Do I have a really crappy attitude?"

- Abdominal pain has many possibilities depending on the location and type of the pain.
- A fever indicates an infection and that the immune system is raising the body temperature above 100.5 degrees in order to kill a virus or bacteria.
- A runny nose is the body's way of trying to dilute allergens or remove viruses and bacteria from nasal passages and sinuses.
- Discharges of any kind have a definite purpose, mostly to remove the offending organism from the area.
- Localized pain can tell us where the problem is.

The advertising media for traditional Western medicine tells us to gain instant relief by making the symptom go away immediately. However, this only masks the message, like putting a piece of tape over that oil light on the dash. In holistic medicine, we recognize that our body wants us to direct treatment toward the cause of the problem rather than blocking and suppressing the symptom.

For example, high cholesterol is a symptom, not a disease. It means there is too much inflammation in the blood vessel walls. We can track the symptom back to its source and eliminate the problem. Once we fix the source of the problem, the symptom will resolve all by itself. Changing how and what we eat, exercising regularly, drinking good water, and avoiding toxins whenever possible are often good ways to fix root causes and therefore eliminate symptoms.

Many over-the-counter and prescription medications suppress symptoms. Short-term suppression is acceptable while we find the root cause, but long-term use of suppressive medications will actually cause more problems. It's better to pay attention to the symptom and fix the underlying cause.

Please understand that sometimes we need modern medicine, but many times we can do things to prevent the need for prescription medications and surgery.

Case Study: MM had severe bone spurs in his neck causing pain down his arm. The spurs were the result of a neck injury fifteen years before. The neurosurgeon was considering surgery. I elected to recommend herbal Hydrangea three times a day and homeopathic

Calcerea Carbonicum 6C once a day at a cost of less than $30. Within three weeks, the neck and arm pain began to subside. He took those two remedies on days 1 through 25 of each month for about six months. Three years later, he is still symptom free. Not everyone is so fortunate, but it is good to try some things first before having surgery.

Author's Note: Herbal medications can lose their effectiveness with long-term use. Taking a "vacation" from the herb for five or six days each month will resolve this issue. We suggest taking the herb on days 1 through 25 if it is going to be used for more than a month.

What works for you: Mechanistic view or vitalistic approach?

Traditional medicine holds a *mechanistic* view of the body, thinking that it is a machine that sometimes needs repair and a doctor to fix it. Prescription medicine might not heal the body, but it will suppress and control the symptoms, and surgery can repair or replace defective parts. The doctor, thinking as a mechanic, focuses on the damaged tissue.

Much of traditional medicine is about suppressing the immune system. Steroids, antibiotics, non-steroidal anti-inflammatories, immunizations, birth control pills, and hormone replacement therapy are all about suppression, not about building the body to make it stronger. Taking these medications generally weakens our constitutional health.

Natural holistic medicine holds a *vitalistic* approach that the body will heal itself. If we listen to the symptoms and can perceive what the inner healing mechanism is trying to tell us, we then can help jump-start the stuck immune system, reset the "thermostat," cleanse the excesses, supplement the deficiencies, remove the obstacles to recovery, and select the correct homeopathic and/or essential oil to correct the current symptoms.

Natural health is about returning to and maintaining our constitutional level of health or building a better "us" than we were when we were born.

Our bodies know how to be healthy. Sometimes, they just need a little nudge. The *vitalist* focuses on helping the body fix things before the damage occurs.

Never well since_____

How many times have you heard someone say, "I have never felt well since I had that _____?" The blank can be filled with mononucleosis, hepatitis, flu, surgery, flu shot, head injury, broken leg, car accident, pneumonia, or any of a host of different things that can happen to us throughout our lives and affect our constitutional health.

Most of the time we totally recover, but sometimes we just do not get completely well. The results can be subtle and of no real consequence or they can be profound and have a huge impact on the rest of our lives.

Many cases of chronic fatigue and fibromyalgia are the result of this problem. Some neurological problems like multiple sclerosis, memory loss, and chronic pain problems might fall into this category.

Traditional medicine has very little to offer people with this situation. Naturopathic and homeopathic medicines, however, have much more to offer. Although occasionally we see an immediate result, most people will see considerable improvement in their "never well since _____..." symptoms in three to six months. If nothing occurs in that time, then the case needs to be reevaluated to look for another remedy.

Many nutritional programs like the Blood Type diet, the Apo E Gene diet, and IgG Food Sensitivity lists help us reduce general inflammation from foods. Supplements like omega-3 fatty acids found in fish oil, cod liver oil, and flaxseed oil are great natural anti-inflammatories.

Homeopathic medicines like Gelsemium and Phosphoric Acidicum have been a great help for people with chronic fatigue after having mono, hepatitis, influenza, or reaction to flu shots.

Homeopathic Arnica and homeopathic Natrum Sulphuricum have worked well for the subtle negative effects of old head injuries.

Homeopathic Phosphorus and homeopathic Cadmium Sulphuricum have been good for the negative effects from surgery, anesthesia, and radiation therapy.

Try some of these things. They have no side effects. If they do not help, then try another until you find a remedy to fix the cause. You will be glad you did!

A little later, I will give you some information on how to select the strength and frequency of a homeopathic remedy.

Why do Christians get sick?

Having been raised in a strict religious community, this is a question I remember asking my mother. She never really had a good answer, but recently I ran across a book by George H. Malkmus titled *Why Christians Get Sick*, and it gave me a bit of insight. The question applies to all religious groups.

The message of this book is "Why wouldn't they get sick?" Most Christians in the United States eat the Standard American Diet (SAD), are exposed to the same toxins, and watch the same toxic elements on television as the rest of the world.

It is my opinion that the source of most physical illness is contamination of our body by food additives, pesticides, herbicides, and heavy metals that are in our food. Toxic material in our water and air, such as volatile organic compounds (VOC), are the other source.

Another source of illness is the contamination of our mental, emotional, and spiritual body by the impressions on the brain by newspapers, television, movies, and other public media.

Isn't it interesting that up until about 30 years ago, it was rare to see cancer, diabetes, heart disease, or other chronic illnesses in wild animals? We saw those diseases in domestic animals but rarely in the wild. Now, we are beginning to see those diseases in wild animals too. The rates of illnesses like cancer, diabetes, heart disease, etc. in humans are all much higher today than 50 years ago in spite of drugs and high-tech modern medicine. In 1900, about three percent of the population was diagnosed with cancer in their lifetime. Now, it is 40 percent for women and 50 percent for men. We are all slowly getting poisoned, regardless of our religious beliefs. I believe that *perfect health* is a cooperative effort between God and us. He gave us the genetics, now we have to do maintenance.

The other answer to this question "Why do Christians get sick?" has to do with how the mind works and what we think about all day long. A few weeks ago in church, we sang a song that went something like this, "Our thoughts are prayers, and we are always praying." I was struck by this concept. We are always thinking, 24/7. What we think about has a huge impact on our health. I will discuss this more later.

The average person showers and does personal hygiene every day, but does not do much in the way of mental, emotional, or spiritual maintenance.

Many Christians and other religious and spiritual people spend some time every day in prayer, study, and meditation, which I think is awesome. However, there is often not enough critical mass of *positive* spiritual thought to totally out-weigh the *negative* programming and media contamination that we receive and then propagate in our own minds. How many times do we run an uplifting song through our head all day long? How many times do we spend the day going over and over the violence we saw in a movie or the argument we had with our spouse or the fear of our current economy? The physical chemistry of our body is negatively affected by the presence of continual unpleasant thoughts. We must learn to change this. A little mental hygiene every day is an excellent idea.

A final factor in the area of religion is that we often pray the problem rather than the solution: "Lord, help me overcome this addiction." Or "Oh, God, what is wrong with my child?" When we focus on the problem and go over it and over it, we create acidic, inflammatory chemistry within our bodies. This might aggravate or extend the situation. Positive prayer, which includes statements of love or gratitude or acceptance, creating a healthy, positive mental picture of what we desire creates less acidic, healthier body chemistry.

In your mind, imagine the outcome as if you already have it, feeling as if it is already done. Then pray this outcome. Remember "pray" is a verb. Do not pray for something, pray it already completed. Let me explain…

Gregg Braden is a well-known researcher and quantum physicist. He has investigated many ancient cultures. Here's an excerpt from one of Braden's book, *Secrets of the Lost Mode of Prayer.* He describes a friend stepping into a medicine wheel to pray for rain during a drought.

I wasn't prepared for what I saw next. I watched carefully as David removed his shoes, gently placed his naked feet into the circle, and honored the four directions and all of his ancestors. Slowly, he placed his hands in front of his face in a praying position, closed his eyes and became motionless. Oblivious to the heat of the midday desert sun, his breathing slowed and became barely noticeable. After only a few moments, he took a deep breath, opened his eyes to look at me, and said, "Let's go. Our work is finished here."

Expecting to see dancing, or at least some chanting, I was surprised by how quickly this prayer began and then ended. "Already?" I asked. "I thought you were going to pray for rain!"

David's reply to my question has been the key that has helped so many to understand this kind of prayer. As he sat on the ground to lace up his shoes, David looked up at me and smiled. "No," he replied. "I said that I would *pray rain*. If I have *prayed for rain* [emphasis added], it would never happen."

Gregg asked, "If you didn't pray for rain, then what did you do?"

"It's simple," he replied. "I began to have the feeling of what rain feels like. I felt the feeling of rain on my body, and what it feels like to stand with my naked feet in the mud in our village plaza because there has been so much rain. I smelled the smells of rain on the earthen walls in our village and felt what it feels like to walk through fields of corn chest high because there has been so much rain."

David had used his thoughts, feelings, and emotions to perceive what he desired as an already accomplished fact. Braden said the following day it started to rain and did not stop until after the rain, itself, had become a problem.

For many years I have taught people to pray the solution, not the problem. We can learn to pray *health*, not *for health* or the removal of the disease. Pray for what you desire by seeing it in your mind and feeling gratitude as if it were already done.

So keep in mind that your thoughts are prayers. So are your actions.

- Monitor your intake of physical toxins in air, food, and water.
- Monitor your intake of media messages.
- Monitor your prayers.
- Monitor your spiritual food.

Intentionally create a positive balance and you will stay healthier, no matter what your religious beliefs.

Depression is often a good thing

For those of us who have suffered with depression, this statement might seem a little cruel, but read on; you will gain a different perspective.

There are several different kinds of depression. I used to have bouts of cyclic depression that would last three or four days. Many have seasonal depression. Then there is reactive depression and finally endogenous depression.

All forms of depression are caused by a reduction of neurotransmitters. These are chemicals made in our brain and by our digestive system. Their job is to help nerve cells communicate with each other to perform a specific task.

The task of keeping our moods stable and on the happy side is a complicated one. What we think about causes certain chemicals to be released and these chemicals determine our mood. Worry and anxious thoughts cause the neurotransmitters to be used up faster than they can be made, and, consequently, this depletion causes us to have the feelings that we call depression.

Feeling this depression is like seeing the red warning light show up on the dash of your car. Its purpose is to tell you something is wrong. In my case, there were certain thoughts and thinking patterns that I had learned in childhood that needed to be updated.

With seasonal depression, these feelings mean you need more sunshine. Melatonin is a chemical that is produced by the pineal gland in the brain when our head is exposed to sunshine and full spectrum artificial light. Fluorescent lights contribute to the problem because they cannot stimulate the production of melatonin. A winter vacation to the sunny south, daily use of a full-spectrum lamp, and 2000 IUs of vitamin D3 twice a day will help.

Reactive depression is part of grief and loss. Homeopathic remedies like Ignatia, Naturum Muraticum, and Pulsatilla have been highly effective in the alleviation of depression related to grief, loss, and abandonment.

Endogenous depression means there is an *internal* chemical imbalance in the brain. This imbalance is usually caused by one of two things: a deficiency in amino acids, like 5-Hydroxytryptophan (5-HTP) or by excessive thinking about old negative situations.

Remember, feeling depressed is a warning. Instead of just taking a medication to raise the neurotransmitter levels, it is better to look for the cause. If you have serious depression and are contemplating suicide, it is time to seek professional help from your doctor or crisis center. Medications might be needed to stabilize things until you can get to the root cause.

Some of us eat because of depression. We have learned that eating high carbohydrate foods loaded with sugars and starches make us feel better due to a temporary spike in blood sugar. It is responsible for much of the fat stored in the abdomen. But remember, we are not camels storing up nutrition for a trip across the desert. We will decrease feelings of depression when we create a food plan that does not include a lot of junk, giving us a more balanced sugar intake, and supplement our diet with vitamins and minerals. Eating only in our eating places—kitchen, dining room, patio, or restaurant—is likely to help remove this habit of eating comfort food on the couch, in the bedroom, in the car, or at the work station.

Likewise, getting rid of the old mental and emotional trash is a must. When we constantly think about some past event, we burn more neurotransmitters than we can make and we begin to have the feeling of depression. A few years ago I bought a new cell phone, but it would not hold a charge very long. I took it back to the phone store. The technician looked it over and said, "Oh, you just have some programs running in the background." That is often the cause of endogenous depression—old programs running in the background.

Another very important component of depression is lack of touch. Being nurtured, being cared for by others, and being touched are essential for our mental and emotional health. When we are lonely and depressed, we need to be touched. Our skin needs stimulation, our scalp needs to be massaged, our hair needs to be combed, we need to be hugged, and we need to be touched. These are not desires, these are needs. Many people come to The Healing Center for a massage; they might think it is for aches and pains, but most of the time it is because they have touch deprivation. Hugging and intimacy are necessary for our health.

Fixing the cause will permanently remove those feelings of depression. Sunshine, full-spectrum lighting, vitamin D3, hypnotherapy, good nutrition, massages, homeopathic remedies for unresolved grief/loss/abandonment issues, essential oils to raise our vibrational frequency, and supplements to naturally restore balance to the neurotransmitters will solve this problem.

Suicide

Vibrant health occurs at three levels: physical, mental/emotional, and spiritual.

Our physical health can be affected directly by physical things such as trauma or infections. It can also be affected by mental and emotional issues. These are called *psychosomatic* illnesses, which are real, physical problems rooted in the emotions. True healing of these physical problems must come from healing the mental and emotional condition first.

When we have issues and challenges that are rooted in the mental/emotional part of us, we sometimes consider suicide. This is actually quite normal because we are genetically programmed to solve problems. When we face something difficult, our brain, just like a computer, will sort through all the possible solutions. Suicide is one solution.

But suicide has a built-in misconception. Because the problem is mental/emotional, the body doesn't need to die. Rather, death needs to come to the mental/emotional idea, old program, trauma, or other misinformation. The only way to create a better life is to release that old "stuff" from the past and move into a new future.

Many years ago during the depths of one of my depression episodes, I contemplated driving my car into a large immoveable object. Then I had the insight that killing my body was not the solution, but I did need to let go of some old, outdated ideas that I thought were true. Hypnotherapy and homeopathic remedies were the ways I used to fix the past and move on into a brighter future.

If you are feeling suicidal and thinking about ways to do it, you must talk to someone immediately. Maybe even medications will be needed for a time. But then begin to search for the mental/emotional traumas that have caused this thinking. When you find them, use tools like Emotional Releasing Letters, Emotional Release Massage, Emotional Freedom Techniques (EFT), hypnotherapy, or some other method to release and remove these misconceptions.

You will then find that suicide no longer comes into your thoughts because the underlying problem is no longer there. The above techniques will be explained in detail later in this book. But, wait, you need to learn a little more first.

It is my belief that our purpose for being here is for our spiritual evolution.

The problems we face help us follow that purpose. When we learn how to overcome the problem, we evolve into a higher spiritual being and become more and more capable of overcoming more and greater things, each of which adds to our spiritual evolution.

Do your mental and emotional housecleaning, love your body the way it is, and enhance your spirit.

Seasonal affective disorder, winter blues, cabin fever

Humans are mammals. Many mammal species hibernate for the winter. This means that everything in the body slows down to conserve energy to get through until spring. In nature this is seen in bears, bats, raccoons, and many other mammals. Ancient man did the same. They would gather food and fatten up all summer and then they would hole up in a lodge, cave, or earth dwelling to survive the winter, only going out if they absolutely had to for survival. There, they did a lot of sleeping. Jane Auel's *Earth's Children* books, including *Clan of the Cave Bear,* are awesome stories that give us insight into some of this winter activity of our prehistoric relatives.

In our culture, we often oppose this aspect of nature. We slim down in the summer because we are more active, and we fatten up in the winter. Instead of listening to our body, we push on through the colder months, working and taking care of life, often not getting enough sleep.

As a result of these natural, genetic, biological cycles, many of us begin to feel the slow down by January or February. Psychiatrists and scientists have named this seasonal affective disorder (SAD) or seasonal depression. Some people call it the "winter blues" or "cabin fever." This simply means some people get a "little nuts" by mid-winter. The medical professionals want us to take medications like Prozac and Paxil, and, yes, sometimes that is necessary for short periods of time.

But there are many other things we can do first. At least eight hours of sleep per day are needed in the winter. Get some sunshine. Actual sunshine is the best because it penetrates the skull and stimulates the pineal gland, increases the production of melatonin and other neurotransmitters. Even a week or two spent in the sunny south in February can fully recharge our solar battery so things do not look so bleak. If you cannot go south, get your head in the sun whenever you do get a sunny day. In the absence of sunshine, tanning often helps, as long as you do not burn and peel. Buy a full-spectrum lamp and place it directly over your head two hours per day. Or you can install full-spectrum fluorescent tubes in your work or home environment to simulate sunlight. Be sure to learn of all side effects before using artificial lamps.

Supplements like 5-Hydroxytryptophan (5-HTP), the amino acid in turkey that makes some people sleepy, can be very useful to improve sleep if taken at bedtime. During sleep, it is converted into serotonin, a neurotransmitter known as "a mood elevator." For some, St. John's Wort is quite good for dealing with the winter blues. Homeopathic Aurum and Aurum Muraticum Natronatum have also proven to be effective for these temporary depressions. Vitamin D3 is highly beneficial. Most of us are deficient in vitamin D and supplementation with 4000 to 8000 IUs per day is recommended if you do not get any sunshine. Vitamin D3 levels should be checked regularly. Ask your doctor to order this.

Exercise is highly important to balance the chemistry and remove sluggish waste products from the body. Find a fun winter activity that will balance out the blues. Make your own sunshine!

Terrain versus germ theory

All of us are familiar with the germ theory, which states that germs cause infections.

So why is it that some people get sick every time something "goes around" and others never get sick? The answer is the terrain theory.

This refers to our body's natural defense system that is constantly looking for and protecting us from problems. If it is not working, we are more likely to become ill.

What keeps the defense system working properly?

- Adequate sunshine, at least fifteen minutes every day.
- Deep breathing and good oxygenation of our tissues.
- Enough good water to keep the urine clear or at least slightly yellow.
- Nutritious "live" foods that contain the enzymes needed to digest that food.

- Functioning bowels, kidneys, skin pores, lungs, and lymphatic system to eliminate waste.
- Consumption of healthy fats, carbohydrates, and proteins.
- Exercise and movement.
- Balanced acidity and alkalinity to prevent inflammation.
- Emotional stability and a spiritual connection to God.

Avoid chlorine, chemical additives, air pollution, which includes smoking, excessive alcohol, sweets, and starches.

So, it is not the presence of the germs and microorganisms that cause illness. It is the state of our body, the internal terrain of our systems that keep us healthy. Dr. Bennett used to say, "Rats won't live in a clean house." This is a great perspective.

Vaccinations

Are you aware of the controversy around vaccinations? We have been conditioned to believe they are necessary and safe, but there are some reasons to think this is not true.

By age 6, a child who gets all of the recommend shots will have received over 75 vaccines. These might contain, as preservatives, mercury, aluminum, gentamicin, and neomycin, which have been accused of causing Asperger's syndrome, autism, and ADD/ADHD.

Most vaccines carry what is called "foreign DNA," which refers to DNA from monkeys, sheep, and chickens used to make the vaccines. Although we are told that it is safe, I am just not sure. It is like finding a fly in your soup.

One other concern is that, by immunizing against specific viruses and not experiencing any of the usually viral childhood illnesses, we are decreasing our society's general immunity against viruses. If this is true, we might become much more vulnerable to a super bug epidemic. It is too late for all of us who have been immunized, but should we keep doing this to our children?

Many health care providers will totally disagree with this information, but many others are beginning to understand the gravity of this situation. You might want to investigate more.

A parent recently asked the question, "Do immunizations cause autism and should we be giving them to our children?"

Vaccines are not the total cause of autism, but I have seen a direct connection in some autistic children. Let me share with you my understanding about what might be happening. In the people I see there is a wide variety, a spectrum. Some people are very sensitive and some people have no sensitivity. The sensitive people react to everything: foods, additives, chemicals, and the like. They can experience a variety of symptoms that range from joint pain, muscle aches, excess nasal mucus, brain fog, anxiety, depression, reactions to drugs and immunizations, and more. These people are also often psychically sensitive and can empathically feel other people's pain and emotions in their own body. On the other end of that spectrum are those who feel nothing and react to nothing. The insensitive ones think the others are crazy. And the sensitive ones feel that no one believes them. Because of this difference in the constitution of people, only some children, the highly sensitive ones, will react negatively to immunizations.

I have been a physician assistant for nearly 40 years and have never seen a single case of measles, rubella, tetanus, polio, or diphtheria. Many would argue that this is because of immunizations, but in countries that do not immunize, these illnesses are not seen either.

I have treated numerous cases of whooping cough and some mumps. This was done very successfully with homeopathic remedies, essential oils, herbal immune boosters, and antibiotics. Read more about this from Dr. Joseph Mercola, DO, at www.mercola.com and Dr. Sherri Tenpenny, DO, at www.drtenpenny.com.

I am not in favor of the heavy immunization schedule suggested by the Centers for Disease Control and Prevention (CDC) and American Medical Association (AMA). Below is the advice I give people who ask, but it should be noted that this is purely my opinion and not an official recommendation. You must research this for yourself and make your own decisions.

1. No infant should be immunized for hepatitis B at birth. Hepatitis B is spread by sexual contact and dirty drug needles. If you are pregnant and an intravenous drug user with multiple sexual partners, then your baby needs a hepatitis B vaccination; otherwise not. It is not good to introduce a totally innocent immune system to an attenuated virus in the form of a vaccination like hepatitis B on the first day of life.

2. The number of cases of tetanus reported in the US every year is less than 50 and the number of deaths reported is less than five. This is not because of immunizations but because of the nature of that infection. Tetanus is an anaerobic organism that lives in the soil, which means it cannot live in the presence of oxygen. It must be introduced into the body by a deep penetrating wound from an object that has been buried underground. So stepping on a nail that has been in the dirt is a high risk wound. Stepping on a nail that has been up in the air is not a risk for tetanus. Even a scratch by a garden tool is not high risk. When we had a predominately agricultural society there were many more cases of tetanus. Today most people never see any true organic dirt.

3. Pertussis (whooping cough) is rare and treatable with antibiotics in the early stage and with homeopathic remedies. I have successfully treated many Amish and un-immunized patients with whooping cough using homeopathic Pertussis, Drosera, Spongea, and Antimonium Tartaricum. I did see one family of four children who had whooping cough. It took three months before they were all recovered and one child was hospitalized for two days. The parents were just worn out, so I can see why most people choose to immunize.
   It is unfortunate that at the present time, single vaccines are not available for all infections. Vaccines are currently prepared in combinations of two or three vaccines. If we had singles, we could choose the beneficial vaccines and avoid the unnecessary ones

4. Diphtheria again is treatable by antibiotics and no health care provider that I know has ever seen a case.

5. Very few cases of polio have been reported in the US over the last 10 years and there are only a few cases in countries that do not immunize. Should we put our children at risk of reactions and autism for such a low-risk condition? It is interesting to note that the US immunization program is credited for stamping out polio

in this country, but all over the world, even in countries where no immunizations were given, there has been a dramatic decrease in polio.

6. A few children have died from chicken pox (varicella encephalitis), but it is very rare. Today, however, there has been a tenfold increase in shingles, which is related to chicken pox, in adults and children. This is because children are getting immunized against chicken pox. This means there are fewer cases of chicken pox so the adults are not getting exposed to that virus and they are losing their natural immunity against the chicken pox/shingles virus (varicella/zoster). There are prescription medications and homeopathic remedies that will shorten the course of chicken pox and shingles infections.

7. Human papillomavirus (HPV) might increase the risk of cervical and penile cancer. The virus is usually self-limiting. The problem with the vaccine, Gardasil, is that it only protects against four of the 200 strains and it appears to have a fairly high rate of serious reactions. I do not recommend this to my teenage female patients.

The reason health care providers are so concerned about not giving immunizations is medical liability. Every year the AMA publishes "The Standards of Care." This document is the treatment bible for traditional Western medicine. If a doctor does not follow those guidelines, he or she can be sued for malpractice. If you do not immunize your son and he dies from chicken pox encephalitis, you could sue the provider. You would not win if the doctor documented that you chose not to immunize, but your lawyer could argue that the doctor should have insisted and that you were not fully informed. The doctors' careers and livelihoods are on the line. Most physicians just simply do not want to deal with that risk when people do not cooperate with the recommended immunization schedule. In addition to that, most of the providers of health care have never even considered that the immunization program is flawed. You are asking them to disregard their basic training.

Every therapy has risks and benefits. You must do your own research then choose for yourself and find a health care provider who will be your coach and support you with good information. But you cannot expect a doctor to put his or her career at risk for your idea unless the doctor also believes as you do.

You can opt out of the vaccine program by signing a waiver, which you can find on Google by searching for "vaccine waiver." But do not opt out until you have researched and know, in your own heart, that you are doing the right thing for you and your child. Your doctor or pediatrician will probably disagree and push to give the immunizations. Be very strong in your convictions and know why you are doing this. Study and trust your intuition.

Personally, I believe the risks of giving flu shots and immunizations to highly sensitive people are too great to justify them. There are natural treatments for all the viral illnesses that currently have recommended vaccines. These are herbal and homeopathic. I will discuss specific natural preventive measures and treatments later in this book.

Chicken pox and shingles

This article is revised from a column by Dr. Mercola.

By giving vaccines, trying to prevent all children from experiencing chicken pox naturally, we might have actually created a *new* epidemic— not in children but in adults, especially elderly adults. There is mounting evidence that vaccinating children for chicken pox could be causing a shingles epidemic. I am seeing this in my own practice in Lakeview, Michigan.

For the vast majority of healthy children, chicken pox is a mild disease without complications. Before the live virus chicken pox vaccine was licensed in the United States in 1995, most children acquired a natural, long-lasting immunity to chicken pox by age six. Less than 100 children died per year from complications of chicken pox in the US.

Chicken pox and shingles are related, caused by similar viruses in the herpes virus family. After a person recovers from chicken pox, the virus can remain dormant ("asleep") in nerve roots for many years unless it is awakened by some triggering factor such as physical or emotional stress. When awakened, it presents itself as shingles rather than chicken pox.

Shingles is marked by pain and often a blister-like rash on one side of the body. Other symptoms can include headache and flu symptoms. Although very painful, most people who get shingles will recover without serious complications and will not get it a second time. However, in people with weakened immune systems, shingles complications can be severe. The most common complication is post herpetic neuralgia (PHN) in which the pain might last for months or even years after the rash has healed. The pain is caused by damaged nerve fibers that then persist and send pain messages to the brain.

Nature has devised an elegant plan for protecting your body from the shingles virus. After contracting and recovering from chicken pox, usually as a child, your natural immunity gets asymptomatically "boosted" by coming into contact with infected children who are recovering from chicken pox. This periodic exposure to the varicella (chicken pox) virus helps protect you from getting shingles later in life.

In other words, shingles can be prevented by ordinary contact, such as receiving a hug from a grandchild who is getting or recovering from chicken pox. But with the advent of the chicken pox vaccine, there is less chicken pox around to provide that natural immune boost for children and adults.

As hard as scientists try to come up with ways to "improve" human biology, they just can't outsmart Mother Nature. By trying to tinker with the natural order of things, we tend to destroy processes that God has masterfully orchestrated to keep us healthy. This dance between chicken pox and shingles is a perfect example.

If you do get shingles, there are both traditional and natural treatments that work well. Many parents are now opting out of the chicken pox vaccine for their children. It is time we think for ourselves and not let the government and the drug companies dictate our health care.

Remember it is not nice to fool with Mother Nature.

Fear: Good and bad

Basic fear is good for us. As children, we learn to avoid pain and seek pleasure. Many times that requires experiencing some pain before we learn to avoid it. It is the fear of getting run over by the car that causes us to wait for it to pass before crossing the street. This is a good thing.

Sometimes, however, our fear gets out of control. When this happens, we can trigger our fight-or-flight response—the release of adrenaline and other chemicals that help us fight the danger or get out of its way—even when there is no physical danger.

The fight-or-flight response is a built-in, automatic mechanism designed for our survival. But if this response is triggered when there is no real danger, we might experience a panic or anxiety attack. An anxiety attack can be manifested into chest pain, heart palpitations, sweating, feeling weak, numbness and tingling hands and feet, and mostly a feeling that death is imminent.

It is important to understand that you cannot die from a panic attack. You might feel like it, but if you can relax and slow down your breathing, the panic will pass.

Learning to meditate can be very helpful for reprogramming old fears that lead to old irrational responses.

Severe fears and phobias can be totally removed with a counseling technique called Neuro Linguistic Programing (NLP). You can look online for NLP practitioners in your area.

Getting adequate sleep and reducing stimulants, sugar, and alcohol are very helpful for lowering the body's sensitivity. Homeopathic remedies like Aconite, Argentum Nitricum, Gelsemium, and Phosphorus all are helpful for this condition. We have found the Bach Flower remedies Mimmulus and Aspen to be very useful for treatment of anxiety and fear. You will learn more about Bach Flower remedies later.

Meridian tapping, Thought Field Therapy (TFT), Emotional Freedom Technique (EFT), and The Happiness Code are other phenomenal ways to deal with fear, and I will discuss this in more detail later.

Bio Energetic Synchronization Technique (BEST), as taught by the Mortor Health System, is another amazing tool for those who experience anxiety.

Don't worry, be happy.

Removing the Obstacles to Recovery

OBSTACLES to recovery are things we do that interfere with our body's ability to heal itself. Learning to remove those obstacles will allow your body to return to its natural vital state. We will lay some groundwork then look at obstacles in the physical, mental, emotional, and spiritual areas.

The hierarchy of therapeutics

Healing takes many forms. Some are medicinal and some are not. It is important to understand these before we continue.

We are most familiar with traditional *prescription* and *over the counter* (OTC) *medicines*. These kinds of medicines force the body into some kind of chemical or cellular change to achieve a certain outcome. They are reasonably predictable and have some side effects. The higher the dose, the stronger the effect until a toxicity level is reached that can be detrimental. For example, Sudafed is a common sinus decongestant that can raise blood pressure and damage the heart.

Herbal medicines are like prescription medicines except the source of the medicine is completely from natural sources and they are not synthetically manufactured. Herbal medicines are like concentrated food. Their function is to "build" when the body has deficiencies and to "cleanse" the body of excesses. Thereby, herbal medicines bring the natural body systems back to normal health. There can still be side effects, but toxicity rarely occurs. For example, herbal hydrangea can dissolve bone spurs and calcium-containing kidney and gallstones, but hawthorn can harm the heart.

Supplements are compounds of natural or synthetic origin that are used to replace or replenish substances that the body can no longer produce or can manufacture only in limited quantity. These are usually intended to "build" in cases of deficiency. For example, vitamin D3 *can be* used to replace missing D3 in sunless Michigan during the winter. Supplements can also have toxic side effects. For example, niacin is an essential vitamin, but too much can raise blood pressure and cause the skin to flush red. Too much vitamin E (more than 400 IU per day) can cause some heart issues.

Tinctures are herbal extractions of the medicinal part of plants that are dissolved into ethyl alcohol. Because they are concentrated, tinctures are usually stronger than the medicinal part of the plant itself, and are usually given in a few drops of water. Tinctures force some chemical or cellular change in the body. When given with care and proper dosing, side effects and toxicities are rare. For example, alfalfa tincture might be used to stimulate appetite in a very ill patient who will not eat. Taking too much would be like eating the alfalfa plant, harmless. However, arnica tincture is highly poisonous when taken internally, whereas topical use is highly beneficial for sprains, strains, and bruises.

This next concept, that of *energy medicine,* is more involved but very important to understand.

Every subatomic particle, every atom, every molecule, every cell, every tissue, every organ, and the body as whole all have a specific resonant vibrational frequency. When our tissues and organs are healthy, they resonate at one vibrational frequency. When they are diseased, the normal vibrational frequency changes to a different rate, usually slower.

Energy medicine refers to natural substances that carry a vibration similar to that of the healthy organ or tissue. When these substances are introduced into the body topically or orally, the healthy frequency can be transferred to the ailing tissue. The normal vibration returns and the illness subsides. This is the principle of harmonics. Remember in harmonics, if you pluck one guitar string, all of them begin to vibrate.

Energy medicine might also refer to the transfer of energy from one person to another for the purposes of healing. The electromagnetic energy from the hands of a healthy person can be transmitted to someone who is ill in order to change the vibrational frequency of a diseased organ or tissue from illness to health. But the receiving party will benefit only if they are receptive to the energy transfer at subconscious levels. "Hands on" healing will be discussed at a later time.

Tinctures, homeopathic remedies, and essential oils can transfer energy to abnormal tissues to change the vibration by harmonics. They cannot force chemical changes in the body; they can only stimulate the body into healing itself. For example, Arnica tincture, homeopathic Arnica, and the essential oil

Lavender are all wonderful for energetically healing sprains, strain, tendonitis, and physical trauma.

In the case of homeopathic medicines, the more diluted the remedy, the stronger its effect. Homeopathic remedies that are diluted more than 24X or 12C no longer carry any of the original physical substance used to make the remedy. This is why there can be no side effects and no toxicity. But even though they have no physical substance left, the preparation still carries the energy signature of the original substance (probably in the digital code of the water used to make the remedy). This energetic effect is strengthened by the dilution and succussion (shaking) process used to make homeopathic remedies. This energy signature can then affect the harmonic vibrations of the diseased organ or tissue, bringing it back to normal. Over 3,000 homeopathic remedies form a complete therapeutic system for dealing with a host of health issues. Homeopathy will be discussed in further detail later in this book.

We can see that there is a wide range of medicinal therapy available to us. It is important to learn more about these and use a practitioner who is knowledgeable in as many levels of therapeutics as possible.

If I knew better, I would do better

A few years ago, a patient said to me, "If I knew better, I would do better." This probably does reflect the situation of many people. Our general health education comes from our parents, health class in school, our friends, health care providers, television, and the internet. Too many times, I see patients who never think about their health until something crops up that causes them to seek health care. My father used to say, "If it ain't broke, don't fix it." In one sense, that is a good attitude. It is not necessary to run to the doctor with every hangnail and sniffle. However, preventive care is a very important part of our overall picture of health.

We all basically know what to do, but sometimes we need a reminder.

Moderation is a key element of life. Many people do things to excess. Begin to develop some common sense. Reduce portions. Drink one or two cups of coffee a day, instead of 20. Drink water instead of pop. Every 20 ounce pop has ten or more teaspoons of sugar (as high fructose corn syrup) in it. If you have one less pop and one more bottle of water per day, you would save yourself 3,600 teaspoons of sugar in one year. Just that would remove, rather than gain, 10 or 15 pounds per year.

Get some healthy fats in your diet. For too many years, we were telling people to eat low fat and low cholesterol. So what did we eat instead? We ate more carbohydrates, starch, and sugars. We need fats to make hormones and the membrane of every cell in our bodies. Fish oil, flaxseed oil, and olive oil are highly beneficial. Be careful not to overheat oils, such as through deep frying, because this will convert them to trans fats, which are very inflammatory to our blood vessels. You will learn more about good fats later.

Limit dairy. For some people, dairy is very inflammatory.

Again, moderation is the key. Alcohol in small amounts has some benefit, but frequent, regular use of alcohol will eventually cause great health problems in nearly everyone. This damage is difficult to fix. The same is true for smoking. The heat and chemicals from smoking do great damage to our lungs. Most of us have an amazing resilience. Many people smoke 40 to 50 pack-years (one pack per day for one year is a pack-year) and still do not have much trouble. Others cannot handle that much smoking because they have a genetically weak system.

All of us have stress in our lives. Sometimes we get overloaded. That is when systems begin to break down. Learning to relax and using some mind coaching or mental training exercises can be highly beneficial.

Pay attention to your body. Learn about your body, attend health classes, prepare yourself, and you will do better.

Muscle response testing

I will use this term frequently throughout this book because we have found it to be a useful tool to find obstacles to recovery. Muscle response testing also known as applied kinesiology can be helpful in food and supplement selection. When I was first introduced to this, I thought it was a bunch of BS. However, over time, I have seen muscle response testing work in many patients with reproducible, dependable results. Most naturopathic doctors (ND) and certified natural health practitioners (CNHP) use this all the time and you can learn to do this yourself.

Remember the word *aura*? It refers to the layers of electromagnetic field that surround our bodies. (In a later section, I will explain this term fully.)

This field has a charge. When you bring something into that field, you will feel attraction or repulsion. Recall how you feel when you meet someone. Some people you could just give them a hug and others make you want to run. This same feeling can be used to select foods and supplements that can be beneficial for your body.

Here is the procedure for muscle testing your own responses:

Stand with feet apart, knees slightly bent. Hold the item in question in front of your heart area. In the beginning do this with your eyes closed. Then just stand there and see if your body sways forward or backward. Generally, if you sway forward (toward the item), it is a sign that it is beneficial for you, but if you fall backward (away from the item), it might be harmful to you. If nothing happens, you may silently make the statement, "This is good for me," and then wait to see what occurs. Movement forward, toward the item is a positive and a repelling motion backward indicates a negative. No movement or swaying side to side is a neutral response and the item in question is likely not beneficial or harmful.

This is called a soft or subjective test, as compared to an objective test like an x-ray or a blood test. With practice, you can become very accurate with muscle response testing, and you can confirm the results through the objective, evidence-based tests of modern medicine.

Before Barb and I opened The Healing Center in 2005, we visited a large number of other health stores and muscle tested many products, using the statement: "This is manufactured correctly." If we got a negative response, we decided not to carry that product in our health store. It turns out this was a very good decision.

Fix it before it is too late

Case Study: Last year, a man came to the office because he could not breathe without supplemental oxygen. He had been diagnosed with pulmonary fibrosis. This is scar tissue and calcium build up in his lungs. He also had a great deal of swelling in his legs. He wanted to know if there was anything natural that he could do to fix this problem. He asked this as he struggled to get air with an oxygen cannula in his nose.

I sat for a moment and stared at him. I was awestruck. Here was a perfectly good body totally broken down, fighting for survival. Was it possible to help him?

Three years earlier, he and I had sat in those same chairs. He had aged at least ten years in just that short time. Back then, he was extremely stressed over some business issues that were causing him to feel great anxiety, worry, and depression. In his attempt to medicate himself, he was drinking alcohol at night until he passed out. Otherwise, he could not sleep. When he woke up, he would have to drink coffee and smoke cigarettes for hours so he could get cranked up enough to face another stress-filled day.

In my notes, I could see that I had prescribed several remedies, but my advice for lifestyle changes had been completely ignored. He was still drinking coffee and Coca-Cola. He said his other doctor told him it was okay. And twice a day, he still had to light up a smoke. Amazingly, he had quit drinking alcohol, but I noticed that he was a little yellow. Sure enough, lab tests confirmed that he had a very sick liver on top of the ruined lungs.

The fact that his heart and kidneys were still doing well is a testament to the tremendous ability of the body to compensate, adjust, and heal itself. But finally, after years of abuse, one or more systems become completely overwhelmed and begin to fail.

This problem begins in the mind. When the financial problems began, he did his best to deal with the problems in the only way he knew. But even when given advice that he asked for and paid for, he was unable to get out of the rat race. Maybe he did not believe that the smoking, alcohol, coffee, pop, and over-eating would eventually catch up to him. Or maybe at some level he really just did not want to live anymore. I do not know.

For this man it might be too late, but maybe it is not. Only time will tell. Can he stop the intake of toxins now? Will he take the recommended herbs and homeopathics? Does he have a strong enough will to live? Is there more on this earth that he still has to do?

Are there lessons he still needs to learn or teach? Only he and God know the answer.

For everyone reading this, please stop for a moment. Think. Are you poisoning yourself in some way? For many of us, myself included, the answer is yes. I love sugar. So, take inventory. Are you damaging your body? Is the situation fixable? If you stopped taking in the toxin, would your life be better? Would you live longer?

For most of us, it is not too late to change. For some, it is and that makes me extremely sad.

Author's Note: About three weeks after the visit that I referred to in the above story, the patient died of cardiac arrest and respiratory failure. It is very sad to see people ruin their lives with the excesses of life, caught in the rat race.

Calling everyone over 40: There is still time!

As people enter the decade of their 40s, I hear them comment that they are getting older.

First, this bothers me a lot because I know what is happening: people are actually programming themselves to get old too soon and die too young. What we think about is what we become. So if throughout our lives we constantly are saying, "I am going to live to be 120 years old," we actually increase our chances of getting to be 100 years old and in good health. When we constantly talk about getting old, it actually accelerates our aging. You know this one by now, "It is not your age; it is just your mileage."

Second, the decade of the 40s is a time when many of us do begin to think about our lives, where we are going, and what we are doing. We may go to the doctor for a physical and blood tests. We might see that we did not take such good care of ourselves. We could realize that an old injury is catching up with us. We sometimes hear ourselves grunting and groaning as we get up out of that chair.

So, now let's analyze our thinking and take inventory of what is going on in our body. Begin programming yourself to live in perfect health until you are 98 or 120. If you need some help with that, you might try my Mind

Coaching CDs, *Coaching for Perfect Health* or *Christian Coaching for Perfect Health*. (See www.thehealingcenteroflakeview.com)

When you do a body inventory, here are some things to ask yourself and think about:

- Are you experiencing any chronic pain?
- Where does that pain come from?
- Do you have any detrimental habits?
- How is that habit hurting you?
- Are you overweight for your height?
- What is the quality of your food?
- What is the size of your food portions?
- How is your energy?
- Are you experiencing the effects of too much stress?
- Do you know how to neutralize stress?
- Are you doing anything that is damaging to your vision or hearing?
- Are your routes of waste elimination (BMs, urine, breath, sweat) working well?
- Do you feel that everything is working the way it should?
- Are you having fun?
- Do you enjoy life?
- Do you love getting up every morning?
- How are your relationships affecting your health?

After you do this little inventory, do some more thinking, such as "What else do I need to know about myself?" "What do I desire to change?"

Most of us have functional health issues that have not yet resulted in pathology or damage. There is still time to fix those issues. Our bodies have remarkable self-healing and compensation mechanisms. So what can we do, what can we learn, how can we heal ourselves, how can we live to be 100+ years old and remain in perfect health? Many have done it, so why not every one?

My mentor Jose Silva frequently said, "I will live to the age of 98 and die in perfect health." And he almost did that, working up until the day he passed over, dying in his sleep at the age of 85, choosing to transition rather than dying because his body wore out.

Start asking, start reading, start searching, educate yourself, take responsibility, and put your health in your own hands.

Physical Obstacles to Recovery

The physical obstacles to recovery include things within our body that affect our physical chemistry and make it difficult for the natural healing mechanisms within us to function correctly.

Toxins

Toxins are any chemical or substance that can cause harm and possibly death to some of the cells in our body. Most of the toxins we are concerned about are the subtle ones that do not cause immediate symptoms. Toxins can enter our body through air, water, food, and our skin. Toxic thoughts are a bigger problem than the physical toxins.

Volatile organic compounds are chemical compounds that vaporize easily. Examples are fumes and vapors like gasoline, paint thinners, perfumes, etc. They enter the body through breathing, the skin, and sometimes contaminated food and water. These often accumulate in our body fat until they are concentrated enough to cause illness. The only way to remove them is by sweating (exercise and sauna), using a cleansing essential oil like Digize by Young Living Essential Oils, and by something called "oil pulling," which I will explain later.

Other toxins enter in drinking water. Bromine, fluoride, and chlorine, because they are chemically similar to iodine, can sit in the iodine receptors on the cells causing sub-clinical hypothyroidism. This means you might experience subtle fatigue, constipation, and skin dryness but still have normal thyroid blood tests. At home, you should have a filter on your shower head and you should drink filtered, pure water. If you drink city water in a restaurant, squeeze a wedge of lemon into the water; this will cause the chlorine to come to the surface and evaporate after a few minutes.

Herbicides and pesticides are often in and on our food. Know where your food comes from and who grows it. Eat locally grown and organic food if possible. Washing food with water and sometimes with enzyme preparations helps a lot, but now some growers are treating some plants systemically and the toxic chemical is inside the food. (See the Dirty Dozen and the

Clean Fifteen in a few pages.) These neurotoxic compounds are stored in our body fat. Removal can be done with cleansing essential oils, foot detox, and exercise.

Growth hormones are often added to plants and animals to increase production and bring food to market sooner. Recombinant bovine growth hormone (rBGH) is used to increase milk production. However, rBGH, although marketed as safe for human consumption, has been blamed for early puberty and menstrual problems in some young women. Steroid growth hormones, which are male hormones to stimulate growth of muscle mass, in beef cattle definitely can cause problems in both men and women. These things are likely culprits in production of visceral adipose tissue (VAT) also known as the "beer belly."

Heavy metals are toxins that are probably present in everyone. Some people feel that our fat sequesters these harmful toxins to protect the more sensitive tissues like the brain and nervous system. Chelation therapy, oral or intravenous, can remove heavy metals. It could be prudent to have the silver-mercury amalgam fillings removed from your teeth. The theory is that mercury oxide vaporizes from fillings that are no longer sealed. This vapor is inhaled and mercury begins to accumulate in body tissues, exerting its effects in sensitive individuals. This is a highly controversial issue in traditional dentistry, so read about it, consult a holistic dentist in your area, and make up your own mind. The best dentists for evaluating this will be those who have trained with Dr. Hal Huggins, DDS, at his clinic in Colorado.

Toxins are subtle, but you can avoid them. Wear a charcoal filter mask when exposed to fumes, drink pure water, wash the veggies, avoid rBGH milk, eat organic food as much as possible, raise your own beef or buy meat from someone you know. Ask them not to add hormones and chemicals to the feed.

If you have had a lot of exposure to toxins, see a natural health practitioner and get some sound information on cleanses that can remove the toxins.

Organic fruits and vegetables can reduce your toxic load

I am passing this information along from Dr. Louisa Williams, ND, author of the book, *Radical Medicine*. We should all read this information.

A 2003 study of Seattle school children showed switching to organic food immediately lowered pesticide levels in their bodies. The study tracked preschool children and analyzed their urine for evidence of exposure to five different kinds of pesticides. Researchers found that children who ate conventional diets had pesticide levels an average of seven times higher than children with organic diets.

A 2006 study conducted at Emory University supported this conclusion. Researchers found that upon switching from a conventional to an organic diet, urinary levels of two organophosphate pesticide metabolites decreased immediately to an undetectable level.

Very few of the families studied ate meals that were 100 percent organic. The researchers defined an organic diet as one that consisted of 75 percent organic foods.

These studies show that making small changes can improve your family's health! Find a Weston A. Price Foundation chapter in your area. They know where to get organic or at least good clean food. www.westonaprice.org. (I will discuss Weston A. Price later.)

The Environmental Working Group, a consumer advocacy and research group, has developed a list of the Dirty Dozen, 12 fruits and vegetables that, when conventionally grown, are loaded with pesticides. They have a free app for your phone to help you select food while shopping.

The group also recommends that you buy the Clean Fifteen, which are fruits and veggies that have the lowest pesticide levels.

The Dirty Dozen: peaches, apples, bell peppers, celery, nectarines, strawberries, cherries, kale, lettuce (iceberg), grapes (imported), carrots, pears

The Clean Fifteen: onions, avocados, sweet corn, pineapples, mangoes, asparagus, sweet peas, kiwi, cabbage, eggplant, papaya, watermelon, broccoli, tomatoes, sweet potatoes

We know that buying all organic is not easy, but begin now and do your best. If you are eating food from the Dirty Dozen list, buy organic. At least they will be less toxic than conventionally grown foods on that list.

The toxic load in our body is responsible for the failure of many of our systems. Blood vessel disease, diabetes, obesity, cancer, Alzheimer's, and others are all related to an excess of toxic material in our body.

Gluten grains

Gluten is a collection of proteins contained in some grass family grains that cause inflammation in some people. The gluten grains are wheat, rye, barley, durum wheat, graham flour, semolina, bulgur wheat, pumpernickel spelt, farina, kamut, and triticale.

Bowel and skin problems, sinus and allergy issues, eye irritations, joint pain and swelling, blood vessel, heart, and artery inflammation, brain fog, and many more symptoms can arise in gluten-sensitive individuals who eat these foods.

Remember that people have a wide range of sensitivities that can change over time. Some are not bothered by anything. Others have extreme sensitivity to everything, including foods, chemicals, medicine, and emotions. And then there are all levels in between. The more sensitive people have more trouble utilizing gluten grains without consequences.

So if you have any issues in these areas and if you think you have inflammation in your body, you might try a gluten-free diet for two weeks. Then challenge your system by eating the gluten grains for one day and watch carefully for the next four days to see if anything unusual is going on within your body. If you get symptoms, repeat this process, which I have named "eliminate, challenge, and observe."

You might be like many people who live in denial of giving up a favorite food. But if the sensitivity reaction happens again, then you are more likely to accept that you might be gluten sensitive.

Because so much of our cultural eating habits are based on grains, we get a lot of exposure, sometimes overexposure. Over time, this excessive exposure can increase sensitivity. The increased hybridization and engineering of wheat seeds have also increased our sensitivity to these products.

The following is a list of alternative grains that you can use instead of the gluten-containing foods: amaranth, arrowroot, buckwheat, chestnut flour, corn flour, cornmeal, flax, millet, oats, potato flour, popcorn, rice, quinoa (pronounced keen-wa, not kwin-o-a), semolina, sorghum, soy flour, tapioca, and teff.

There is some controversy over some of these. Oats might have some gluten contamination from processing in machinery that also processes wheat products. Some classify semolina as a gluten grain and some say that spelt is gluten free. It is best to muscle test these and then use the "eliminate, challenge, observe" protocol mentioned above.

There is also a condition called celiac disease. People with this situation usually have bowel and skin problems related to the intake of gluten grains and casein, the protein in milk and dairy products.

Gluten sensitivity and celiac disease are two different things. Celiac disease is diagnosed by biopsy of the stomach lining and a blood test that is called anti-tissue transglutaminase antibodies (tTGA). Read below for methods of testing for gluten sensitivity.

Testing yourself for food sensitivities

There are two kinds of allergic reactions: immediate and delayed. We don't usually test for immediate reactions because we know what they are by your immediate reaction. Testing for delayed reactions can be done with skin scratch or intradermal tests and with a blood test called a radioallergosorbent test (RAST). This is the test done by most traditional allergists. It looks for immunoglobulin E (IgE) antibodies and immediate, permanent allergic reactions.

Delayed sensitivities that can react up to four days after eating a food cause the greatest difficulty. These reactions can be tested by a method called enzyme-linked immunosorbent assay (ELISA), which looks for immunoglobulin G (IgG) antibodies. The symptoms associated with delayed sensitivities are usually very subtle. They include increased nasal and bronchial mucus, fatigue, joint pain, muscle aches, brain fog, skin reactions, abdominal pain, constipation, diarrhea, irritable bowel syndrome (IBS), inflamed bladder or interstitial cystitis (IC), and much more. It is important to know that IgG sensitivities will gradually disappear with avoidance of the offending food. The ELISA testing for delayed food sensitivities can be arranged by contacting your local natural health care provider.

The "eliminate, challenge, and observe" protocol is also a way to test yourself for food sensitivity. I mentioned this before in relationship to foods that contain gluten, but it needs to be repeated here. To conduct this test, simply eliminate a food group for two full weeks. Then challenge your system by eating foods in that group for one day. Then observe for four days without eating additional food in that group. Watch for a difference in symptoms, comparing the day before the challenge to the days during the observation period. These symptoms might be subtle or dramatic. They could be immediate or delayed up to four days.

A second method to test yourself for food sensitivities is called the "Pulse Test." Begin by eliminating the food group that you wish to test for 48 hours. Then sit at rest for ten minutes while distracting your mind with passive activities such as reading or watching a movie. Then check your pulse and write it down. Then eat the test food and check your pulse again five minutes and ten minutes later. An increase in pulse of more than ten points indicates a reaction. This would be considered a subtle, yet immediate reaction. You should then go on to the elimination testing to see what other symptoms emerge.

The five most common foods that cause delayed sensitivity reactions are dairy products, wheat and gluten grains, corn, eggs, and yeast/mold/fungus foods. The last food group contains the following foods: mushrooms, foods that are raised (bread and pastries), foods that are aged (meats and cheeses), and foods that are fermented (alcohol, vinegar, sauerkraut).

Doing a cleanse

Most of us are full of toxins. Therefore, *everyone* should do some cleansing, but not too often. People with chronic diarrhea should not do cleansing without supervision by a doctor or other health care provider who is familiar with the process. At The Healing Center, we have mostly used products made by Nature's Sunshine Products (NSP) and Young Living Essential Oils. We have chosen these because they have an excellent reputation for quality. There are many other reputable companies. If you are not sure, muscle test the product to see if it energetically matches your system.

A colon cleanse is a good general thing to do. We like TIAO-HE Colon Cleanse by NSP. A liver cleanse is good to restore liver function. We suggest Liver Cleanse Formula by NSP. Some colon cleanses also cleanse the liver, so check the label. Kidney Activator by NSP is good for—you guessed it—the kidneys. Mega Chel and Heavy Metal Cleanse by NSP remove toxic heavy metals like lead, mercury, etc. A candida cleanse can help clear the body of excess yeast and fungus. Aerobic exercise (breathing and sweating), sitting in a sauna, using an essential oil like Digize from Young Living, and oil pulling (see Tonics later in this book) are good ways to cleanse volatile organic compounds (VOCs) like benzene and toluene. These come from gasoline, air pollution, paint thinner, perfume, etc. and are stored in your body fat.

Cleanses need to be followed by a period of building tissues before doing another cleanse. Remember, in natural health, we are either cleansing the toxins and excesses or building the tissues by replacing deficiencies.

Drinking plenty of chlorine-free water is absolutely necessary to cleanse efficiently and correctly. To determine the appropriate quantity of water, use the general guideline of one third to one half of your body weight in ounces, up to a maximum of 100 ounces per day. If you weigh 180 pounds, then drink 60 to 90 ounces per day, but no more than 100. This is a guideline only, so do not become obsessed with getting exactly this amount of water. Make sure to observe the color of your urine every time you use the toilet. It should be clear or light yellow. If it is dark, you need more water. We will talk more about water shortly.

Don't be concerned that this cleanse will act like a massive laxative. That's not how it works. It acts by healing the membranes of your colon at the cellular level so that wastes, toxins, and unwanted chemicals that are removed from the liver and body fat can be discharged down the toilet instead of being reabsorbed back into your blood.

If you are highly sensitive or have a very toxic colon, it is possible that you might get very loose bowel movements. If that happens reduce the dose and follow up with your health care provider. Always begin with less than the recommended dose for a few days to see how you respond.

These cleanses should not be used for children or someone who is very weak or has a serious illness such as Crohn's disease, colitis, or cancer. Cleansing is not suitable for people with anorexia or bulimia. When in doubt about how this will affect your overall health, consult your doctor or other qualified natural health practitioner.

Case Study: JG, a 48-year-old woman, had been diagnosed with Alzheimer's disease. This lady was very sensitive, mostly to volatile organic compounds (VOCs). She and her husband had completely renovated their home, removing all the plastic, plywood, vinyl tile, and other things that were giving off VOCs. By doing this and doing some cleansing of her internal organs, she functioned quite well.

Then one day, she ran into a large department store to pick up some photos. When she came out, she was unable to find her way home. I believe that the chemicals in the air from all the products and plastics in the store "intoxicated" her. This lasted for about three days. She continued to have extreme environmental sensitivity, but is getting better and better as she continues to detox using a variety of methods.

Water

Water is essential for a healthy body and your cells cannot work at their maximum efficiency if they are dry. Yet, most people are chronically dehydrated. Remember, your cells should be like grapes, not raisins.

Remember to watch your urine color. It should be clear to slightly yellow. If it gets dark, you are becoming dehydrated. When you first start drinking a lot of water, you will notice that you will urinate more frequently. This will change after a few weeks. It takes a while to rehydrate all those raisins.

The best water is pure. Well water is good if it is tested for and proven to be free of harmful trace minerals and toxins like agricultural and industrial wastes. Drinking city water should be avoided if it has been treated with chlorine. Chlorine kills the good bacteria in your system and might be harmful to some cellular functions. It might also interfere with the iodine receptors on the cells of the thyroid and lead to sub-clinical hypothyroidism. If you must drink city water, add some lemon, and then let it stand a few minutes. This will help the chlorine rise to the surface and evaporate off.

Some bottled water is not very good. The best are filtered and ozonized for purity. It's hard to know how the water has been processed, but you can read the labels and buy only water that shows no additives. Bottled water should not be heated or frozen in the bottle. Under these temperature extremes, some of the chemicals from the bottle leach into the water. The plastic might act as a xeno-estrogen, which is much stronger than human estrogen and can create a host of symptoms associated with too much estrogen (more on that later).

Soft water might have a lot of salt in it. Drinking it regularly is really not very healthy, especially for people with high blood pressure.

Flavored water should be avoided. The constant use of empty carbohydrates (artificial sweeteners) will cause your carbohydrate digestion mechanism to stop working. Then when you do eat sugars and starches, the mechanics to deal with them will be sluggish and not function well. There is much evidence that shows an increase in appetite and urges for sweets within 30 to 60 minutes after consuming any of the artificial sweeteners.

The best water is steam distilled or filtered with reverse osmosis (R/O). You might want to add a mineral supplement if you are drinking distilled water all the time.

Drink plenty of pure water with your meals. I was taught to limit water with meals to avoid diluting digestive enzymes, but I now disagree. Water helps liquefy the food for better digestion and assimilation. Avoid soft drinks completely, but especially with your meals.

Room temperature water is best. Water that is too cold will slow down some cellular functions. If you have a sluggish metabolism already, cold water might contribute to the issues of belly fat. Drink plenty of pure water every day.

Routes of elimination

As our bodies take in air, water, food, and sunshine, energy is produced to sustain our lives. But there are waste by-products of this energy production. An example of this would be uric acid that is produced when we break down red meat. There are also wastes that are toxic material that we took in but cannot use. A good example of this would be aluminum that we get in pop cans, foil, cookware, worn Teflon coated pans, and antiperspirants.

So how do wastes get out of our body? Most elimination is through our liver and colon. The liver processes our blood, removing harmful wastes. These wastes are moved into the small intestine through the bile ducts and then to the colon for elimination from the body with our bowel movements. Adequate amounts of pure water and fiber are crucial to make this system function properly.

Next, a very large amount of waste is cleaned out of our body through the kidneys in the form of urine. Blood is filtered through the kidneys, which removes the water soluble wastes. Much of the water that we drink every day goes through this urinary system, carrying with it loads of waste. You would not flush out your car's radiator with soda pop or coffee, would you? Use water!

The third route of elimination is the respiratory system, the lungs. Carbon dioxide is removed with every breath we exhale, but so are other aromatic compounds. Bad breath is an example of waste that is not being removed through the bowels and kidneys and is coming out through the lungs. Regular deep breathing and aerobic exercise keep the lungs working well. Adequate water is again very important for proper lung function.

The last route is through the skin, which produces sweat and skin oil. Many waste materials are part of the sweat and oil. Body odor tells us that the other routes of elimination are not working fully. Blocking sweat with under arm antiperspirants is a very unhealthy practice. It is acceptable to use deodorant, but avoid the antiperspirants. Let them see you sweat. If you change what you eat, drink lots of water, cleanse the colon, and take your omega-3 oils, you will be amazed that you really do smell good naturally. Yes, I know it is hard to believe, but a healthy body does smell good, much like a healthy baby.

Estrogen

In the last few years, we have heard a lot about estrogen increasing risks of breast cancer, uterine cancer, and blood clots. As a result, many women have stopped using hormone replacement therapy.

Unfortunately, many of us, both men and women, are still getting too much estrogen. Hydrocarbons have estrogenic effects on our body. Called xeno-estrogens, these are by-products of fertilizers, pesticides, fumes from oil products, off-gases from plastics (the funny smell in your car when it sits in the sun), and soft plastic containers. The xeno-estrogens are much stronger than what our body makes, and they will often block the estrogen receptor sites on our cells. Estrogens, called phyto-estrogens, are also found in soy products. Avoid products that have soy isolates on their labels. However, whole organic soy products are acceptable. And finally, the visceral adipose tissue (VAT), the big belly, can become a huge source of unwanted estrogen because the fat produces an enzyme, aromatase, which converts testosterone to estrogen.

Women with too much estrogen experience weight gain, mood swings, anxiety/depression, insomnia, weepiness, abnormal pap smears, uterine fibroids, breast tenderness, migraines, foggy thinking, and gallbladder problems.

Men with too much estrogen have thinning hair, low sex drive, prostate enlargement, irritability, breast enlargement, abdominal weight gain, headaches, and erectile dysfunction.

We cannot really totally escape the influence of these chemicals, but we can reduce them. Ideally, we should eat organically grown food or at least home grown food. Avoid sprays and commercial fertilizers. Wash your fruit and veggies before eating them. Consider using Nature's Fresh enzyme spray by NSP to break down herbicides and pesticides found on fruits and vegetables. Use hard plastic or glass food storage containers. Drink good water from glass or stainless steel bottles. Use glass and stainless steel for cooking and heating.

Women might need to use progesterone cream to balance the excess estrogen. I suggest you read the book *What Your Doctor Won't Tell You about Hormone Replacement Therapy* by Dr. John Lee, MD.

Hormone Balance Tests

Take the little test below, shown here with permission from Dr. John Lee (See www.johnleemd.com for more information), to see if you have any hormone imbalances. This will help you decide if you need to have physical testing.

Saliva or blood tests can also be used to determine hormone deficiency levels. Then natural hormone creams can be prescribed to balance some of the hormone issues. I prefer the saliva test over the blood test because of lower cost and the accuracy is very similar.

HORMONE BALANCE TEST FOR WOMEN

Symptom group 1

___ Cyclical headaches	___ Insomnia
___ Early miscarriage	___ Painful, lumpy breasts
___ Anxiety	___ Infertility
___ Premenstrual syndrome (PMS)	
___ Unexplained weight gain	

Symptom group 2

___Vaginal dryness   ___ Night sweats
___ Painful intercourse   ___ Memory problems
___ Chronic bladder infections   ___ Lethargy
___ Depression   ___ Hot flashes

Symptom group 3

___ Puffiness and bloating   ___ Abnormal pap smear
___ Rapid weight gain   ___ Breast tenderness
___ Mood swings   ___ Heavy menstrual flow
___ Anxious depression   ___ Migraine headaches
___ Insomnia   ___ Foggy thinking
___ Red flush in face   ___ Gallbladder problems
___ Weepiness

Symptom group 4

___ Weepiness   ___ Insomnia
___ Early miscarriage   ___ Painful, lumpy breasts
___ Unexplained weight gain   ___ Cyclical headaches
___ Anxiety   ___ Infertility
___ Puffiness and bloating   ___ Abnormal pap smear
___ Rapid weight gain   ___ Breast tenderness
___ Mood swings   ___ Heavy menstrual flow
___ Anxiety or depression   ___ Migraine headaches
___ Foggy thinking   ___ Red flush in face
___ Premenstrual syndrome (PMS)
___ Gallbladder problems

Symptom group 5

___ Acne   ___ Unstable blood sugar
___ Thinning hair on head   ___ Infertility
___ Ovarian cysts   ___ Mid-cycle pain
___ Polycystic ovarian syndrome (PCOS)
___ Excessive hair on face/arms

Symptom group 6

___ Debilitating fatigue   ___ Unstable blood sugar
___ Foggy thinking   ___ Low blood pressure
___ Thin and/or dry skin   ___ Intolerance to exercise
___ Brown spots on face

If you checked two or more items in any one category, please go to the hormonal imbalance in the appropriate categories below.

HORMONE IMBALANCE

Symptom group 1: Progesterone Deficiency

This is the most common hormone imbalance among women of all ages. You might need to remove inflammatory foods from your diet, get off synthetic hormones, including birth control pills, and possibly use progesterone cream.

Symptom group 2: Estrogen Deficiency

This hormone imbalance is common in menopausal women, especially those who are petite or slim. You might need to remove inflammatory foods from your diet, take women's herbs, and add a little bit of natural estrogen.

Symptom group 3: Estrogen Excess

In most women, this is usually solved by getting off the conventional synthetic hormones.

Symptom group 4: Estrogen Dominance

This is caused when you don't have enough progesterone to balance the effects of estrogen. You can have low estrogen, but if you have even lower progesterone, you can exhibit symptoms of estrogen dominance. You might need to take a liver cleanse, which will increase your body's ability to remove the excess estrogen, or you could use a bio-identical progesterone supplement. This is covered later in this book and in great detail in Dr. John Lee's book, *What Your Doctor May Not Tell You About Menopause.*

Symptom group 5: Excessive Androgens (Male Hormones)

This hormone imbalance is common in women who have poly-cystic ovarian syndrome (PCOS). This is most often aggravated by too much sugar and simple carbohydrates in the diet. You should get your blood sugar and insulin tested. Low carbohydrate diets are very helpful. Some women do need prescription medications such as Metformin. Consult your health care provider if you fit in this symptom group.

Symptom group 6: Cortisol Deficiency

This hormone imbalance is common in women who have tired adrenals, which is usually caused by chronic stress. If you are trying to juggle a job and a family, chances are good you have tired adrenals. You might need to take an herbal combination like Adrenal Support from NSP.

Read Dr. Lee's book so you understand these ideas better.

HORMONE BALANCE TEST FOR MEN

Symptom group 1

___ Weight loss	___ Enlarged breasts
___ Loss of muscle	___ Lower stamina
___ Lower sex drive	___ Softer erections
___ Fatigue	___ Gallbladder problems

Symptom group 2

___ Hair loss	___ Headaches
___ Prostate enlargements	___ Breast enlargement
___ Irritability	___ Weight gain
___ Puffiness/bloating	

If you checked two or more items in any one category, please go to the hormonal imbalance in the appropriate categories below.

HORMONE IMBALANCE

<u>Symptom group 1: Testosterone Deficiency</u>

This is hormone imbalance is most common in men over the age of fifty. You can remedy it with special nutritional supplements, increased muscle building exercises, and supplemental hormones, including dehydroepiandrosterone (DHEA), androstenedione, and natural testosterone. You can find details in Dr. John Lee's book *Male Hormone Balance for Men.*

<u>Symptom group 2: Estrogen Excess</u>

This hormone imbalance is most common in men with large abdomens. You can balance excess estrogen with one of the natural male hormone supplements, muscle building exercise, weight loss, not cooking in plastic, and reducing inflammatory foods in your diet and not eating any foods that contain soy or phyto-estrogen.

Hormone replacement therapy (HRT)

As we get older, our ability to produce hormones steadily decreases. For this reason, hormone replacement therapy (HRT) has been a big deal in health care for many years.

A hormone is a chemical substance manufactured by an organ in the body and released into the blood that then causes some action on other cells or target organs. An example is the thyroid stimulating hormone (TSH), which is made by the brain and stimulates the thyroid gland to make thyroxin, which is another hormone that controls many other processes in the body.

HRT usually refers to artificially replacing hormones that are missing because of aging, surgery, infection, immune disorders, etc. These are usually estrogen, progesterone, testosterone, and DHEA, which are present in women and in men, and replacement might be helpful for both sexes.

In women, one use of estrogen is to prepare the female body for pregnancy. If pregnancy does occur, progesterone is then produced in large amounts to support that pregnancy. When these two hormones are out of balance in a non-pregnant woman, there can be many symptoms, depending on the imbalance. One of the conditions is called estrogen dominance, which includes fatigue, migraines, mood swings, panic attacks, depression, fibroids, fibrocystic breasts, fluid retention, miscarriages, infertility, irregular cycles, severe menstrual cramps, and heavy menstrual flow.

After menopause, many women experience hot flashes and other very uncomfortable symptoms. These are due to hormone imbalances.

For many years, health care providers prescribed hormone replacement therapy, using medications like Premarin and Provera. For many women, this did relieve their symptoms. But in 2002, the results of a study called The Women's Health Initiative found that these hormones markedly increased the risks of breast, uterine, and ovarian cancer in those taking the HRT.

The problem was that these prescription HRT medications were not exact matches for the naturally occurring hormones made by the body. Hormones and other natural products that are exact matches cannot be patented and the big pharmaceutical companies rarely spend money developing a product that cannot be patented. Some of these medications were synthetically made in a laboratory and some were extracted from the urine of pregnant horses. Because these hormones did not exactly match the body's natural hormones, the target organs often were not affected in the expected or desired way, sometimes causing immune system responses that could lead to inflammation, scar tissue, cysts, and cancers.

The solution to this problem is bio-identical hormone replacement therapy (BHRT). Bio-identical simply means that the hormones used to treat the imbalances are exact matches for human hormones or they stimulate production of the missing hormones within our own tissue, like the adrenal glands. These hormones are made from plant sources, and they are exact matches to the hormones made by our body, therefore the risks of cancers are no greater than expected.

Simple saliva tests costing about $150 can determine the exact hormone deficiency. Blood testing can also be done, but is much more expensive (around $600) and no more accurate. We have found that over the counter progesterone cream has been effective for many women. If that does not correct the imbalance, a prescription cream made from natural ingredients can be created by a compounding pharmacist.

In addition to feeling much better, most women who use BHRT have improved bone density and actually lower their risk of cancer, especially if they change from traditional HRT to the bio-identical products.

Liver

The liver is a large organ found in the right upper part of the abdomen and is considered to be part of the digestive system. It has many functions. Some of these functions are linked to the workings of the gallbladder, which I will discuss in the next section. The liver is vital for good health and a long life.

Our liver handles all the incoming nutrients from the digestive tract. As things are absorbed from the small intestine, they are transported to the liver by the portal system. In the liver, the nutrients are separated into useful and harmful.

The good stuff is further processed to be used for energy or stored for future use. The harmful stuff is sorted out and sent to the bile ducts, which collect bile to be stored in the gallbladder. In the gallbladder, these wastes are combined with bile salts. These are then discharged whenever we eat something with fat in it. The gallbladder contracts and pushes the bile out into the common bile duct, then into the small intestine. Here, in the small intestine, the bile salts assist in digestion of fats. The wastes can then be discharged out of the body with a bowel movement. If the colon is functioning properly, these wastes will not be reabsorbed back into the blood.

Meanwhile, back in the liver, the food is being processed into usable energy and stored for future energy. The liver is an important component of maintaining health blood sugar. When the liver is not functioning well, it sometimes needs some help in the form of a liver cleanse. This does not mean going out Saturday night and drinking a dozen beers. It means taking some herbs to clean out the little canals where all the chemical reactions of the liver occur.

Use an herbal liver cleanse every three to six months, depending on how toxic you are and how much you have abused your liver in the past. Abuse of your liver is not just excessive use of alcohol, but also things like use of multiple prescription medications, exposure to toxic material in a work environment, being overweight, and experiencing frequent emotions of anger, rage, and bitterness.

Gallbladder

As many of you know, we can live without a gallbladder. It is best to keep it if you can. However, sometimes the gallbladder gets diseased and has to be removed. So what is the gallbladder and how do we keep it healthy?

The gallbladder is a sac attached to the hepatic ducts, which collect bile as it is made by the liver, and to the common bile duct. The gallbladder stores the bile until it is needed it to help with digestion.

Bile has many things in it, mostly waste material that the liver has cleaned out of the blood. One of the components of bile is bile salts. When we eat something with fat in it, a signal is sent to the gallbladder to contract it. This squeezes some of the stored bile into the small intestines. The bile salts help the fatty food mix with the rest of the watery material you have eaten. It acts like a detergent to help the water and fat to mix.

Over the last 30 years, the medical community has been telling people to avoid fats. As a result many people have more gallbladder problems because there is not enough stimulation of the muscles in the gallbladder. We need to eat good fats, especially plant fats, like olive oil. Most of us should have two tablespoons of virgin, cold-pressed olive oil or coconut oil every day.

When people drink more pop, tea, coffee, and juices while having less water, we see chronic dehydration as a factor in poor gallbladder function and the formation of gallstones.

Most people do not know that surgery might not be needed if gallstones are present. Most gallstones are made of compacted cholesterol. Herbal hydrangea will help dissolve calcium-based gallstones. Gallbladder Formula by NSP will help soften and dissolve other types of gall stones. The gallbladder can also be flushed out. Do this by eating nothing but raw apples, applesauce, apple juice, fresh pears, or pear juice and water for two days. This will soften any stones if they are made of cholesterol. At the end of the second day, mix 2 to 4 ounces of lemon or grapefruit juice with 2 to 4 ounces of olive oil in a blender. Drink it before it separates. Then go to bed and lie on your right side as much of the night as possible. You might have some cramping and some abdominal discomfort. If you have stones or a sluggish gallbladder, you should be able to see stones or sludge in your bowel movement in the next day or two.

Author's Note: Precaution. It is rare, but this gallbladder cleansing process has been known to push stones into the cystic duct or common bile ducts where they can get stuck. If this occurs, you might need to have surgery to clear those stones. In nearly 20 years of recommending this protocol, I have never seen one stone get stuck. Do not do this if you have an infected or diseased gallbladder. The weak, damaged tissues might not be able to contract adequately to push out the stones. You might want to consult a naturopathic physician or holistic health care provider before doing this gallbladder flush. Your regular doctor probably is not aware of this procedure because the allopathic standard of care for gallbladder disease is surgical removal.

If your gallbladder has been surgically removed or is congenitally absent, you do not get the benefit of bile being injected into the small intestine when you eat a fatty meal. The bile just drips directly from the liver into the duodenum, which is the first portion of the small intestine.

Most people who are missing their gallbladder do just fine without it, but some have pain and indigestion or diarrhea after meals. Digestive supplements, such as the enzyme lipase and ox bile, taken with the meal artificially assist with the emulsion and digestion of fats to fatty acids. If you have chronic diarrhea, add fiber or take a prescription medication called cholestyramine (Questran) to bind up some of the excess bile salts that could be irritating the lining of the small bowel. Discuss this with your doctor or health care provider.

Case Study: FM was a man in his late 50s. He came to see me because he was losing weight and having diarrhea 10 to 15 times a day. Otherwise, he felt well and there was nothing else in his history except that his gallbladder had been removed 20 years before. I could have done a bunch of tests but elected instead to have him use food enzymes with ox bile and lipase. That helped but not enough, so we added prescription cholestyramine powder, ½ to 1 packet once per day in the morning. This combination totally cleared the diarrhea and his bowel movements became normal, one or two times per day.

To keep your gallbladder healthy, drink plenty of water, eat good fats, especially from plants, and flush the gallbladder every six to 12 months.

Deep breathing

Twenty-five years ago, I took some relaxation classes. We were taught about deep breathing.

If you ask someone to take a deep breath, usually they will lift their shoulders and expand the ribcage filling the lungs. While this is good, deep breathing using the diaphragm is better.

Instead of raising the shoulders and ribs, push out the abdomen as far as you can. When you do this, you bring down the diaphragm. Breathing this way provides several benefits.

First, deep breathing improves oxygenation to all cells, which in turn improves their function.

Second, deep breathing with the diaphragm improves movement of lymphatic fluid that fills the space between cells. This fluid carries all the waste products from the cells. Muscular motion and vibration pushes this fluid upward into the chest where it collects into the thoracic duct, which drains the fluid back into the veins. When the lymphatic fluid does not move properly, we feel fatigued and listless.

Third, deep breathing helps with blood flow in the veins. The aorta, which is the large artery that carries blood to the lower half of the body, and the inferior vena cava, which is the large vein that returns blood back from the lower half of the body, pass through the diaphragm. The aorta is a high-pressure system, and usually blood flows easily through the opening in the diaphragm. The vena cava is a lower-pressure system and sometimes, if the diaphragm is not moving adequately during breathing, the blood flow in the vena cava through the opening in the diaphragm can be restricted. This will create back pressure in the veins that might cause liver congestion, varicose veins, and hemorrhoids. Sometimes the excess fluid in the veins is pushed out into the tissues, causing swelling in the legs or collection of fluid in the abdominal cavity.

Everyone, especially those bothered by liver problems, leg swelling, varicose veins, or hemorrhoids, should practice deep abdominal breathing for three to five minutes three times every day. The procedure is simple. Caution: Heed this gentle warning—start slowly!

How to breathe deeply:

- Wear loose fitting clothing.
- Sit or lie down because breathing deeply could make you dizzy. Inhale deeply through your nose, pushing out your abdomen. Then try to inhale more, lifting your shoulders and ribs.
- Next, exhale through pursed lips or with a big sigh. Exhale as far out as you can.
- Now repeat this, inhaling and exhaling continuously for 30 to 60 seconds in the beginning.
- Gradually work up to three or even five minutes per day.
- If you become light headed or dizzy, stop and rest.
- The next day, do a little more.

In case you didn't notice, deep breathing happens naturally with aerobic exercise, so that would be a good plan too.

Deep breathing prior to meditating improves the depth and clarity of your meditation.

If you love gadgets, use an incentive spirometer to more objectively measure your ability to take in deep breaths. This device is commonly used in hospitals to ensure that patients are breathing deeply enough after surgery and while bedridden.

Digestive enzymes

Americans love to eat. One of the causes of poor health is that we do not digest and absorb our food well. We might be overweight but yet starving.

Digestion begins in the mouth. Adequate chewing is very important. Please do not do the "chew, chew, swallow" thing like most Americans in a hurry. Remember what your mother said, "Chew your food at least thirty times." It was good advice then and still is today. In the mouth, enzymes begin to break starch down to glucose, which is the basic energy unit for our body.

In the stomach, hydrochloric acid (HCl) converts pepsinogen into pepsin, which is needed to break down large proteins into smaller units called polypeptides and peptides. Many of us do not have enough HCl for the following reasons: we take acid blockers for gastro esophageal reflux disease (GERD), we are over 50 years of age, or we eat too much at any given meal. So in many cases, our proteins do not digest well, which can cause symptoms of GERD.

In the small intestine, bile from the liver and gallbladder is added to the food you have just eaten to help break up fats. From the pancreas, digestive enzymes are added to the mix. Amylase breaks down starches and complex sugars to glucose; lipase breaks down fats to fatty acids; and protease breaks down polypeptides and peptides to amino acids. When this entire process works correctly, the smallest possible units—glucose, fatty acids, and amino acids—are then absorbed for nutrition, energy, body building, etc.

Again, if we eat too much at any one meal, there might not be enough enzymes to go around, and there could be a lot of undigested food just hanging around. When the large food components, fat, carbohydrates, and proteins are not broken down properly, several things can happen. Some undigested food gets absorbed into the blood, leading to the development of food allergies and auto-immune disorders. Some of it moves on into the large bowel.

In the large bowel, undigested food can feed bacteria, yeasts, and parasites. It can also ferment, leading to gas, bloating, abdominal pain, and re-absorption of wastes into the blood. This causes bad breath, body odor, irritable bowel syndrome, and chronic fatigue, not to mention the embarrassing gas. The unmentionable foul smelling gas is a definite indication of poorly digested foods that are being putrefied (not petrified) by yeast and bacteria, leaving behind the bad odor. Smaller portions of food at mealtime, supplemental food enzymes, probiotics (good bugs), and a colon cleanse will usually clean up this toxic waste site.

Fruits and vegetables naturally contain the enzymes the body needs to break down the components in food. Raw or lightly steamed fruit and veggies are the best because the cooking process has not had a chance to destroy the natural enzymes. Canned and over-cooked foods have no natural enzymes left in them. Meats, dairy, and grains do not contain these enzymes, so cooking them actually improves the digestion process. Just an aside here: people with inflammatory bowel disease (like colitis or Crohn's disease) and chronic diarrhea should cook all vegetables and fruit. Raw fiber can mechanically scrape the lining of the intestines, adding to the inflammation.

Foods without additives are better, so select and prepare food properly and eat small portions. If needed, adding a good digestive enzyme at the beginning of a meal is one way to regain and maintain digestive health. Make sure the supplement contains hydrochloric acid, usually listed as Betine HCl, cellulase, protease, pepsin, lipase, and amylase so it can help in the digestion of fiber, carbohydrates, fats, and protein.

Remember the saying, "We are what we eat?" I like to change that to, "We are what we eat and can assimilate." That means our body has to be able to break the food down properly in order to use it.

Human genes and our DNA do not control life

Since the 1950s, we have been taught that our genes and DNA control everything about our body and our health. We hear a lot about genetic illness, genetic causes for everything from breast cancer to diabetes. I hear all the time, "It is in my genes. I cannot help that I am fat." Well, that is not true. There might be family tendencies, but there is more than simple genetics at work here.

Research brought to light by cellular biologist Dr. Bruce Lipton, PhD, in his book *The Biology of Belief* gives us quite a different view of how biological life is controlled. It turns out that the only true genetic conditions are referred to as congenital birth defects. The rest of our illnesses are not controlled directly by our genes.

Our body contains over 100,000 types of protein, which led the creators of the worldwide human genome project to think that the human body, which is relatively large and complex, would have a comparable number of genes. When the project was completed, they were very surprised to find that we have only about 25,000 genes. In comparison, a fruit fly has 18,000 genes, and a simple earthworm has 24,000 genes. If it were true that our genes controlled everything, we certainly would need more genes than a worm or a fruit fly.

So it became apparent that there is another controlling mechanism that tells the 25,000 genes how to make more than 100,000 types of protein. That other controlling mechanism is the cell membrane, the covering for every cell in our body. This membrane is made of fats and proteins arranged in a sandwich much like an Oreo cookie. Embedded in this cell membrane are specialized proteins called receptors and effectors. The receptors sit idle until they get a signal from outside the cell. The receptor then activates an effector, which activates a gene to make a certain protein. So it is these signals that control things.

There are three sources or origins for the signals:

- the chemical environment around the cell
- toxins from outside the body
- thoughts from the mind

The *chemical environment* is controlled by the quality and quantity of food and drink we consume, how much sunshine and water we get, and our emotions.

The *toxins* are controlled again by what we eat, what we inhale, how well we eliminate wastes, and how much exercise we get.

The *thoughts* part is very interesting. Most of our thoughts are automatic recordings that have been programmed into us by parents, friends, media, teachers, doctors, ministers, and other people in general. Some of these old programs come from childhood experiences of fear and anxiety. Some of them are factual and some are misconceptions. For example, if even a bright child is told that he or she is stupid, that inaccurate thought signal might inhibit the receptors and effectors that stimulate mental activity in the forebrain. And the child's intelligence could, consequently, be reduced.

Mental house cleaning is very important if we want to remain healthy and productive our whole lives. Learning to meditate is one of the best ways to update the old programs and misconceptions. This process of consciously reprogramming our genetics is called epigenetics, and we will be hearing much more about that later in this book.

Artificial sweeteners

The brand name products Equal, Splenda, and NutraSweet are common artificial sweeteners that many of us use on a regular basis. Their generic names are saccharin, sucralose, and aspartame, respectively. These products are very unhealthy for a variety of reasons.

Equal has been known to significantly increase the chances of bladder cancer. Splenda has a lot of chlorine in it that will kill the good healthy bacteria in our digestive tract and might promote yeast overgrowth in the bowel and vagina. Chlorine also competes for the iodine receptor sites on the cell membranes in the thyroid, which can cause clinical hypothyroidism even if the thyroid blood tests are normal. NutraSweet, as it is broken down, produces small quantities of formaldehyde, which is very inflammatory, damaging to all tissues, and difficult to eliminate from the body.

The more damaging problem with these sweeteners is their effect on blood sugar, increasing the risk of diabetes and obesity. Whenever we eat sweet or starchy carbohydrates, the pancreas produces insulin. The insulin is supposed to assist with the transport of the sugar into the cells so it can be used for energy. But because these artificial sweetener products have no carbohydrate value, the insulin cannot be used up, causing significant increases of insulin in tissues. This excess insulin actually causes inflammation and damage to cell membranes, to insulin receptors, and to the inside of the blood vessel walls. This is a cause of insulin resistance in type 2 diabetes.

Constant use of carbohydrate-empty sweeteners will cause the body's carbohydrate digestion mechanism to become sluggish or stop working. Then when you do eat sugars and starches, they are stored instead of being burned for energy.

There is evidence that when we use artificial sweeteners, we experience an increase in appetite and carbohydrate urges within 30 to 60 minutes afterward. Daily use of these products can cause as much as ten pounds of weight gain per year.

It is much better to use pure cane crystals, raw honey, pure maple syrup, unsulfured molasses, or stevia. These are safe, much healthier, and taste good. They will improve your health and reduce the risk of further damage to your tissues.

High fructose corn syrup (HFCS)

Fructose is a five carbon sugar found in many plants. The food industry found that this sugar was easy and economical to extract from grains like corn, it had high sweetness content, and it was easy to transport in liquid form. It has become the standard sweetener in food for many years.

After reading an article by Dr. Mercola, I decided to share some of the information. You can read the whole article online at www.mercola.com. It is a great site, but just be aware that it is quite commercialized. Here is part of Dr. Mercola's message.

New research shows that there are big differences in how the sugars fructose and glucose are metabolized by your body. Overweight study participants showed more evidence of insulin resistance and other risk factors for heart disease and diabetes when 25 percent of their calories came from fructose-sweetened beverages instead of glucose-sweetened beverages.

Fructose is a five carbon sugar and glucose is a six carbon sugar. Sucrose, which is table sugar, is one fructose and one glucose molecule bonded together. We have enzymes in our bodies to break down glucose to be used for energy. We do not have the ability to easily break down and use fructose.

A study looked at 32 overweight or obese men and women. Over a 10-week period, they drank either glucose or fructose sweetened beverages totaling 25 percent of their daily calorie intake. Both the groups gained weight during the trial, but imaging studies revealed that the fructose-consuming group gained more of the dangerous belly fat that has been linked to a higher risk for heart attack and stroke. The fructose group also had higher total cholesterol and LDL cholesterol, and greater insulin resistance.

This is not the first study showing that fructose harms your body in ways glucose does not. Two years ago, another study concluded that drinking high fructose corn syrup, the main ingredient in most soft drinks throughout the world, increases your triglyceride levels and your LDL cholesterol. And, just like this latest study, these harmful effects only occurred in the participants who drank fructose, not glucose.

Today, 55 percent of sweeteners used in food and beverage manufacturing are made from corn, and the number one source of calories in America is soda pop, in the form of high fructose corn syrup. Corn syrup is now found in every type of processed, pre-packaged food you can think of. In fact, the use of HFCS in the US diet increased a staggering 10,673 percent between 1970 and 2005, according to a recent report by the USDA.

Ironically, the very products that most people rely on to lose weight, low-fat diet foods, are often those that contain the most fructose, cause the most weight gain, and a craving for more of the same!

Fructose from fresh fruit is not a problem because it contains fiber and enzymes. These help us digest and use the fructose instead of store it as fat. Fructose, without its natural enzyme, must be processed by the liver. While the liver is doing that, it cannot process any other carbohydrates. Because of this bottleneck in the processing system, many of the other carbohydrates that we have eaten at the same time as the fructose get stored as fat instead of being used for energy. So get rid of the high fructose corn syrup.

Eliminate processed, prepared, boxed foods. Cook and bake from scratch. Use honey, pure cane crystals, pure maple syrup, apple sauce, stevia, and xylitol for sweetening.

You will be amazed at how good you feel and you will easily eliminate unwanted pounds, especially the unhealthy belly fat.

Earlier, I presented a case study about a "sweet little boy" who became a temper-tantrum tyrant, controlled by high fructose corn syrup. This is happening to countless children. It might be happening within your family. Think about it.

"Supersize Me"

You probably have noticed that McDonald's no longer uses the "Supersize Me" slogan in their marketing. After the documentary movie *Supersize Me* by Morgan Spurlock came out in 2004, we became much more aware that not only the quality of food but also the quantity of food was responsible for the growing problem of obesity in this country. In the movie, Spurlock ate three times a day at McDonald's for 30 days. He gained 27 pounds and his cholesterol went from a healthy 180 to 240. He developed a fatty liver with liver enzymes that looked like that of an alcoholic. He actually became addicted to the fast food, and it took him about 18 months of eating a healthy diet to recover.

We know it was not only the trans fats in the food but also the high carbohydrate load and the quantity of food eaten that created the problems. If you hold your palms together to make a small bowl, that is the quantity of the entire meal that you should place into your stomach at any one time. Your body does not make enough enzymes to digest more than that at one time. If you eat a larger amount, the excess passes, undigested, into the small bowel and becomes fuel for the bad bugs that hang out there. This turns the digestive track into a toxic waste dump, causing bloating, foul-smelling gas, and reflux.

The average American man eats 100 hamburgers per year. The average Big Mac is about 550 calories (the measure of heat/energy in a food) and a Burger King Whopper is 770 calories. If you add a regular Coke and large fries to that, it could add up to 1200 to 1400 calories per meal. That is the amount of food that some people should eat in one whole day. If you eat one hundred meals like this per year, it could equal an annual weight gain of about 15 pounds. As a general rule, 100 calorie reduction per day will equal about 10 pounds eliminated per year.

When you eat out at a restaurant, if possible, avoid deep fried food, especially French fries. Consider eating a smaller sandwich instead of the big one. Better yet, have a small salad with a small amount of dressing or good olive oil with pepper and spices added for great flavor. When Barb and I eat out, we often split a meal. We are both satisfied and do not feel that over-stuffed feeling associated with eating large portions. Have water with lemon instead of the soft drink. Avoid the all-you-can-eat special deals. Remember, "Slimmer Size Me."

At The Healing Center, we use an amazing hypnosis technique called The Virtual Gastric Band. This was created by Sheila Granger, a hypnotherapist from the United Kingdom. Graduates learn to automatically select smaller portions because they feel full faster. See the Virtual Gastric Band section in coming pages.

Milk is for baby cows

Before I begin, let me extend my apologies to the dairy farmers. I grew up on a dairy farm, and I understand how milk and dairy products have become a huge part of our culture and a huge industry in our country. However, from a natural health point of view, there are a lot of problems associated with the use of milk and dairy products. Wouldn't it be great if the American Dairy

Association, the milk producers and natural health advocates would work together to find a solution to these concerns?

One of my old teachers used to say, "Milk is for baby cows." What he meant was that humans are the only mammals on the planet who drink the milk of another species. We are the only mammals who continue to drink milk after we get teeth and are weaned. About the time we get teeth, our digestive enzymes begin to change so we can digest foods other than mother's milk.

People often ask, "If I do not drink milk how will I get my calcium?" I ask back, "Where do cows get calcium?" The answer is, "From the grass they eat." We should be getting our calcium from our food, especially green vegetables—just like cows do. And we can use supplements, if needed.

The issues with milk include:

Lactose intolerance. This means that some people do not make lactase, which is the enzyme that digests milk sugar. If that is missing, the milk sugar (lactose) goes undigested into the small intestine, causing diarrhea, cramps, and gastro-intestinal upset.

Casein. This is the protein in milk. There are two types of casein: A1 and A2. Many people are sensitive to A1 casein. A2 casein, which most people can handle, is found in the milk of most goats and Jersey or Guernsey cows. Every child with recurring ear infections, asthma, and allergies should be tested for delayed sensitivity to dairy, which often causes respiratory problems.

Lectin. Lectin comes from the left-over components of the immune system of the plants and animals that we use for food. Based on our blood type, lectins can cause inflammation that will create problems in our genetically weakest system.

Xanthine oxidase. This is an enzyme that is released in free form during the process of homogenizing milk. In its free form, this enzyme is highly acidic, and any of the calcium benefits from drinking milk are used up trying to buffer the acidity of this unbound enzyme.

Osteoporosis. The three countries with the highest dairy and beef consumption are United States, Australia, and Sweden. And they have the most incidences of osteoporosis. Any connection? Yes, calcium from our bones is depleted because it is used to neutralize the acidity of meat, coffee, black tea, sugar, starches, processed milk, and other dairy products such as aged cheeses.

Use the "eliminate, challenge, and observe" method I described earlier. Try going dairy-free for two weeks, then consume some dairy and see what happens in your body. If your body doesn't react within four days, then it's apparently okay to continue with dairy in your diet. But continue to monitor your body for possible dairy-related issues in the future.

The pulse test also works. Consume no milk products for 24 hours. Then sit at rest for five minutes, check your pulse, then drink milk or eat some dairy product. Check your pulse at five and ten minutes. If your pulse goes up ten points or more, you are experiencing a reaction.

Case Study: One of our pediatric patients with ADHD had a pulse change from 74 to 128 after one glass of milk.

Experiment. See if milk might be harming you.

Raw milk: The sacred food?

In primitive cultures, milk products, especially butter, were referred to as a sacred food.

It was given to both parents before conception and to the woman during pregnancy and while nursing. Because those cultures did not have refrigeration and raw milk spoiled easily, all of these cultures used some form of fermentation to preserve milk products. These included yogurt, sour cream, cottage cheese, and other cheeses. When made from unprocessed milk, these foods can be very beneficial.

Let's discuss the problems with processed milk, that is, milk that is pasteurized and homogenized.

During the process of pasteurization, milk is heated to 161 degrees to destroy the bacteria that are supposedly harmful to humans. This heating causes a great deal of damage to the natural benefits of milk. The proteins are modified, the natural enzymes are damaged, good healthy organisms are destroyed, and some healthy fats are changed to trans fats that are inflammatory to our tissues.

During the process of homogenization, a powerful enzyme called xanthine oxidase, which was embedded in the butter fat, is released. In raw milk, this enzyme kills pathogenic bacteria, but when broken out of its natural environment, it is extremely acidic, foreign to our body chemistry, and no longer able to kill the bad bugs. This enzyme is one of the contributing causes of osteoporosis and arterial inflammation.

Weston A. Price was a dentist who did a huge amount of research in 1920s and '30s into primitive cultures. He provided the world with very solid information about the use of dairy products for the health of teeth and bones. His book *Nutrition and Physical Degeneration* is well worth reading. The Weston A. Price Foundation carries on his work and can be helpful to locate raw dairy resources. One of their websites, www.realmilk.com, should give you chapter locations as well as the date and location of their annual convention.

If you cannot tolerate dairy products, neither raw nor processed, don't cry. There are good alternatives. We recommend rice milk, almond milk, rice yogurt, coconut yogurt, rice ice cream, almond cheese, and organic goat cheese. While traveling in Egypt, Barb and I ate camel ice cream and had no problems.

We generally do not recommend commercially produced soy products, unless they are certified organic and made from whole soy. Soy isolates have been known to be very inflammatory and might contain phyto-estrogens, which are plant-based estrogens that are not healthy for males, growing children, or women who have estrogen dominance and weight issues.

Please note that since butter contains no milk sugar and no milk fat, it is acceptable and actually beneficial to most people.

Sleep, rest, and relaxation

Lots of us do not know what these words mean.

A few years ago, I had some patients who worked for a company that required them to work 12-hour days, seven days a week. Some of their employees began to experience fatigue-related problems. Many had mental and emotional problems. Others had social and marital difficulties. The rate of accidents and injuries was higher than average.

Sleep deprivation studies have all shown dramatic reduction in human performance when we do not get enough rest. Initially, loss of sleep causes daytime fatigue, then irritability, then neurotic behaviors of anxiety and depression, and finally psychotic behavior and hallucinations.

This is because humans are designed to need recuperation time.

During rest and sleep, many of the body's processes shut down. The chemicals that we used up during the day are replenished.

We have all heard that we need eight hours of sleep per day. I think that varies quite a bit from person to person. Some need ten and some can get by with six hours.

I do not think that all the hours need to be at the same time. I have an acquaintance who writes books. He goes to bed at 9 pm and gets up at 1 am. He then writes for four hours and returns to bed at 5 am for three hours more sleep. This works very well for him and he does not experience any tiredness or fatigue during the daytime.

If, for some reason, you do not get enough sleep at night, you can augment your sleep with power naps or cat naps. This kind of nap should be limited to 15 minutes or less. The reason is that most rejuvenation occurs in the first stages of sleep. If you sleep longer, you will awaken from a deeper stage of sleep and will feel more fatigued than rested.

Many of our religious traditions teach us to rest on the Sabbath. That is a day for spiritual reflection and rejuvenation, but it is also important to spend that time resting and recharging our physical body as well. That does not mean to do absolutely nothing; it means rest and recreation. To recreate is to re-create or rebuild yourself, physically, mental, emotionally, and spiritually. Every person should take personal time to be alone and rejuvenate the body, mind, and spirit.

Insomnia

Unfortunately, some of us have difficulty sleeping. To go to sleep, we must relax completely physically and mentally.

Physical insomnia can be caused by pain, dehydration, muscular tension, restless legs, and the inability to relax the muscles. Homeopathic Rhus Toxidendron and Arsenicum Album are good for physical muscular restlessness. Magnesium 250 to 750 mg at bedtime helps the muscles relax. Although too much magnesium can cause diarrhea with a laxative effect; if that happens, reduce the dose.

Progressive relaxation can be helpful. Start at the top of your head. Tighten your scalp and facial muscles, then relax them. Do the same with your neck. Slowly go down your body, progressively tightening and relaxing all muscle groups.

Mental insomnia is characterized by an overactive mind that will not shut down. The mental pictures get brighter, sharper, and faster. Your self-talk becomes faster and louder. Stimulants like caffeine, tobacco, worry, anxiety, grief, and stress can cause the mind to go into overdrive.

What you eat before going to bed definitely influences your ability to sleep. Homeopathic Moon Drops, Herbal Sleep, 5-HTP, melatonin, homeopathic Ignatia, Arsenicum, adrenal support herbal combinations, and several other natural remedies can help with mental insomnia.

New studies show that sleeping in a dark room is important. So turn all the lights off or wear an eye mask.

Highly sensitive people should unplug all electronic devices to avoid over-stimulation from electromagnetic field vibrations and remove crystals from their sleeping rooms.

There is a nice mental exercise you can use to train yourself to go to sleep. This was taught to me by Jose Silva, and it is part of the Silva Method of Mind Development and Stress Control.

1. Get into bed, ready for sleep
2. Find a comfortable position.
3. Take three deep breaths.
4. Do progressive relaxation from head to toes.
5. Then imagine you are standing in front of a large chalkboard, chalk in one hand, and an eraser in the other.
6. Imagine drawing a large circle and slowly draw a large number 100 in the circle.
7. Then mentally, slowly erase the number 100 being careful not to erase the circle. It is important to mentally draw and erase very slowly to train your brain to slow down.
8. Then to the right and outside the circle write the word sleepy.
9. Next draw a large number 99 in the circle.

10. Then slowly erase the 99, careful not to erase the circle.

11. Now trace over the word sleepy.

12. Continue this, each time decreasing one number until you go to sleep.

The first night it might take a while, but the next night will be better. Keep doing it each night until all you have to do is take the three deep breaths and off to sleep you go. Some people find that playing white noise and classical music can be very helpful to facilitate this process.

Plastics: The convenient poison

It seems like we are always pointing out the bad stuff that can harm us. We also point out the options and alternatives.

When we stray from nature, we increase our rate of harm from ingestion of toxic substances. Our body has an amazing ability to adjust and compensate. Eventually the accumulation becomes too great and some part of the body fails, creating serious effects.

I recently read an article in "Johns Hopkins Cancer News" about the use of plastic food containers. Storage containers and water bottles should be high-density polyethylene (HDPE). This will show up as a "7" in the recycling triangle on the bottom of the container. Cooking and heating should never be done in plastic containers. Stored food should be removed from them and heated in glass or stainless steel cookware.

The problem is that soft plastics—those with less than a "7" recycling number—leach toxic by-products into the water and food. Cooking in plastic accelerates this process. Dioxin comes out of the plastic into the food and enters our system. We have a hard time eliminating these fat-soluble toxins, so we store them in our fat, which keeps the toxins away from more sensitive tissues like the brain and nervous system. This could be a reason why some people have difficulty eliminating undesirable weight. Sweating, deep breathing, and use of some essential oil can cleanse some of those toxins and make it easier to eliminate fat and lose weight.

Use glass or stainless steel containers for cooking and heating. Use HDPE #7 glass or stainless steel for water bottles.

The chemical process involved in heating food with a microwave oven creates free radicals. In scientific terms, free radicals are molecules that are missing an electron in their outer shell. Much like your car when it is missing a tire, these molecules do not function the way they should. Eating foods containing free radicals causes inflammation in our bodies. This can lead to damaged arteries, irritated joints, allergies, asthma, irritated bowel, and other maladies.

Barb and I use the microwave for heating hot packs but never for cooking. So we recommend that you also never use a microwave for cooking.

If you must use a microwave, place the food on or in a glass container and cover it with a paper towel instead of a plastic wrap. Paper cups are better than Styrofoam, which is a form of plastic; although some paper containers are lined with plastic.

Be observant. Please teach your children about microwave cooking. We old dogs are already contaminated, but only for the last 30 years or so. Our children will have much more exposure, so they have to be much more careful.

Sunshine

Earlier, we talked about maintaining a healthy terrain to prevent illness. Here is a little more detail on that subject.

Did you ever see a plant that has not gotten enough sunshine? It is long, spindly, and weak. This occurs because the plant is not getting the full spectrum of color it needs from sunshine. Similarly, detrimental things occur in humans who do not get enough sunshine.

Several studies have been done in large office buildings where people are under fluorescent lighting, instead of sunshine, most of the day. There are increased illnesses, more stress and mental problems, lower productivity, and more mistakes compared to people getting adequate sunshine.

The full spectrum of sunlight is needed for humans to maintain health. Vitamin D3 is manufactured in our skin by exposure to sunlight. This powerful hormone regulates calcium, bone metabolism, and as many as sixty other body functions. Vitamin D3 is now thought to be an important cancer preventer.

Fifteen to thirty minutes of exposure to sunshine, three times per week is generally adequate for vitamin D3 production for most humans. This should be done before 10 am and after 3 pm to reduce skin cancer risks. It seems that this is enough sunshine to make enough vitamin D3 to prevent deficiency, but it is probably not enough to help overcome some conditions like osteoporosis.

A simple blood test can determine if you have enough D3 in your system. Our experience now with testing a lot of patients shows that most people are deficient in vitamin D3.

The current recommended daily allowance (RDA) for vitamin D3 is 400 IUs per day. Research shows that 4000 to 8000 IUs per day divided in two doses is more likely the needed amount, especially for women, the elderly, and those who are chronically ill or take a lot of medicines.

Later in this book, I write about the Budwig Support Tonic. This program calls for a daily intake of flaxseed oil mixed with low-fat cottage cheese or yogurt for the prevention and treatment of cancer. It is interesting to note that vitamin D3 and flaxseed oil both have the same resonant vibrational frequency as sunlight. This means that when we are exposed to sunshine, all the vitamin D3 in our body that came from supplements is activated as if it were made by the sunshine. It also means that the lipoprotein cell membranes that came from the essential fatty acids in flaxseed oil will also be activated, thus increasing energy and improving oxygen carrying ability.

Sunshine also penetrates through our skull and stimulates the pineal gland in the center of the brain to produce melatonin. This is one of the serotonin hormones that acts as a mood elevator and helps with healthy sleep. With lack of sunshine, we might get seasonal depression, winter blues, and cabin fever in the wintery north. That is why we feel better on a sunny day, why a week or two in the sunny south in February fixes the winter blues, and why some of us just feel like hibernating in the winter.

So enjoy the sun carefully or use a full-spectrum lamp at home. You could replace your regular fluorescent bulbs with full-spectrum bulbs if you are stuck in a closed space all day.

Exercise: Why we need it

One of the dangers of learning new information is that it sometimes requires a major shift in our thinking. Many people resist this and continue to think in their old ways even though, in the back of their minds, they know their thinking is flawed. Over the last few months, this has happened to me, and I am doing my best to maintain my new information rather that sliding back into the old thought pattern.

From Pam McDonald's groundbreaking work *The Perfect Gene Diet*, we have recently learned that the Apo E Gene controls how the body transports fats. We also know that each of the six Apo E genotypes is influenced by different types of food and different types of exercise. This means that many chronic diseases are caused by a mismatch between the body's genotype preference and the actual food intake and exercise activity that a person has been doing.

This means that counseling patients on lifestyle changes can be very precise if we have the Apo E genetic information. Now I find myself feeling handicapped when I do not have that information. So I have had to revert back to some sort of generic directions that will have to be satisfactory until my patient gets a genetic test.

Exercise has been a topic that I have tried to ignore for most of my career. This was not based on the unimportance of exercise but my own dislike for what I thought was useless expenditure of energy and a waste of time. However, with some new understanding, I am changing my thinking.

There are two factors that have affected my way of thinking. The first has to do with the need for muscle. I recently attended a conference on chronic illness and chronic liver disease. Some research was presented that showed a Frailty Score that determined survival probability. The most important feature of evaluating survivability after an accident, acute illness, or surgery was the amount of lean muscle mass a person carried. The exact mechanism of this is not yet clear. However, the indications are that, if we can build and maintain muscle mass, we can reduce frailty and enhance how we deal with chronic illness, acute illness, injuries, and surgery.

The second factor has to do with normal body weight. We know that resting muscle uses only stored fat as its fuel source. Working muscle uses glucose, stored glycogen, and protein as its fuel. Three hours after eating, we have either stored or burned everything we ate in that meal. If we do not eat again for a period of time beyond three hours, we begin to break down the protein of our muscle and use it for energy, thus weakening our muscles.

Some time ago, I wrote an article titled "It is good to feel hunger – You are burning stored fat." It is apparent now that this concept is not accurate.

True biological hunger tells us when it is time to eat. But it is important to think of food as fuel and to fuel our body with healthy food, not junk.

Each meal and snack must contain some fats, proteins, and carbohydrates. If we remain hungry and do not eat, the body will begin to "feed on itself." It feeds on stored sugar (glycogen) and on our lean muscle. The down side of this is that reducing the total muscle mass ultimately reduces the consumption of stored body fat, thus reducing our ability to eliminate excess fat.

So, these two things go together. We need to exercise to build muscle and eat every three hours to maintain that new muscle. Only then can our weight normalize.

Exercise: Aerobic and anaerobic

We need both aerobic and anaerobic exercise.

Aerobic exercise is hot, sweaty, fun activity that gets our heart rate up and our blood pumping. This can be walking, biking, running, swimming, dance, Zumba, mini trampoline … anything that gets things moving.

This type of exercise has a minimum rate to benefit our body and a maximum rate that reduces risk of damage to heart and blood vessels. This heart rate range is determined by age.

Target Heart Rate ranges for aerobic exercise

Age	Target HR Zone 60-85%
20 years	120-170 beats per minute (bpm)
30 years	114-162 bpm
35 years	110-157 bpm
40 years	108-153 bpm
45 years	105-149 bpm
50 years	102-145 bpm
55 years	99-140 bpm
60 years	96-136 bpm
65 years	93-132 bpm
70 years	90-128 bpm

Anaerobic exercise consists of stretching and strengthening without maintaining a sustained elevated heart rate. Examples of this type of exercise are yoga, soft forms of martial arts, weight lifting, walking, or the use of a vibration plate. Anaerobic exercise is important for tendon, ligament, and joint health as well as building muscle and maintaining our balance.

Both aerobic and anaerobic exercises build muscle. On the following pages, we will explore what this means and how much we should do of each kind of exercise. In the meantime, get moving. We were designed for motion and mobility, not sitting and riding.

Exercise: How can I get out of doing it?

I am still trying to avoid exercise because my old programming has always been, "I hate exercise," and, "working out is a waste of time." But now, I have been doing it and, each day, it is getting easier.

Gradual transition into an exercise routine is very important. In the past, I would go out the first day and do too much. I recall several occasions of having good intentions for exercise and quitting because I hurt so much the next day. Slowly working into this process is very important.

In 2011, Barb and I studied with Pam McDonald, author of *The Apo E Gene Diet*. Based on the results of my Apo E Gene test and Berkley Heart Lab's advanced cardiovascular markers, I now know that I need a lot of aerobic exercise. For my genotype, toxins cannot be removed from my body very easily through my kidneys, liver, and bowel; they need to come out through my lungs and skin. The aerobic pathway is the only way these poisons can be removed from a body with my genotype. That means aerobic exercise; hot, sweaty, fun activities are a must if I want vitality and longevity.

My former thinking would be to dream up ways to get out of exercising. I might even have gone so far as to subconsciously arrange for a sprained ankle or other injury. This time, I am motivated. My genotype has a high probability of neurological disorders, like Alzheimer's and multiple sclerosis. These diseases are caused by intake of toxins that we cannot eliminate, which means that, consequently, they accumulate. This causes malfunction of the nervous system, much like a plugged oil filter or too many dead leaves clogging a rain gutter's down spout or like a nice trout stream being turned into a stagnant swamp.

The solution to the problem of accumulated toxins that must come out through the lungs and skin has three parts:

1. Eat the correct foods and stop adding to the toxic load in your body.
2. Improve the detoxification process and clear out existing accumulations by exercise that produces lots of sweat and deep breathing.
3. Add an essential oil like Digize from Young Living that will break down pesticides, VOCs, and other fat soluble toxins into compounds that can be easily removed from the body through the other routes of elimination.

The good news is that our miraculous body can heal itself if we do not continue to promote the obstacle to recovery. I am amazed when I see how we constantly poison ourselves, eating for pleasure, eating chemical additives, and then expect to remain healthy. We put all those toxins into our body, don't do anything to clear them out, and expect our doctor to fix us when we get ill. I know. I have been there myself. I used to drink six diet Cokes a day, smoke my pipe, drink too much alcohol, and sit around watching television all night. Ten years ago, I made some big changes, but now it is time for more.

My choice is to have forty or more years of health. So that means I need—and desire—to exercise. Both aerobic and anaerobic.

Maybe you can exercise on your own. Maybe you need a personal trainer. Maybe you need to join a fitness facility. If you're not sure about your genetic preferences, divide your exercise time between half aerobic and half anaerobic. Whatever your preference, just do it!

Exercise: Start slowly

As with any change, when starting to exercise, start small. Your seemingly insignificant, moment-to-moment choices will lead to big results over time. Here is an example.

Case Study: SD was 33 years old and 50 pounds overweight. Reading about an acquaintance who was running a half marathon, she joked that she could never do that. Yet, she did want to eliminate some weight. Her sister was getting married in nine months, and she would like to be smaller for that occasion. So she had motivation.

She started by driving her car around the neighborhood to map out a one-mile walking route. She received professional instructions to walk that mile three times over the first two weeks then twice in the following week. She was soon up to walking it four times each week. Then she began to jog 20 steps, then 30, then 50, then 80.

Each day, she added a small change until she was jogging half a mile, then a whole mile, then two miles, then more. Over six months, she gradually moved up. She eliminated 50 pounds of body weight and has now run four full marathons.

This is a good example of how small, seemingly insignificant choices every day will lead to amazing results over time.

Superbrain Yoga

Superbrain Yoga is a simple and effective technique to energize and recharge the brain. It is based on the principles of subtle energy and ear acupuncture. This powerful technique is explained in Master Choa Kok Sui's latest book *Superbrain Yoga.*

Pilot studies on the effects of Superbrain Yoga on school children with disabilities such as ADHD/ADD, developmental and cognitive delays, Down's syndrome, and specific learning disabilities showed significant increase in academic and behavioral performance, greater class participation, and improved social skills. In one study, the result of an electroencephalograph showed increased amplitude in the parietal-occipital region of the brain. This indicates that the exercise leads to increased brain electrical activity. This exercise seems to be very helpful for adults as well as children. Best of all it can be done in three minutes per day. Here are the steps:

Step One: Face the sunrise. This form of yoga should be done in the morning, so that your concentration and focus will apply throughout the whole day. If you do not know in which direction the sun rises in relation to your room, wake up a little earlier than normal and watch before doing your yoga. Do not fret; this will work facing any direction.

Step Two: Remove any earrings. With your left hand, grasp your right earlobe with your pointer finger and thumb. Make sure that the thumb is facing away from you.

Step Three: With your right hand, grasp your left earlobe with your pointer finger and thumb. Once again, make sure that your thumb is facing away from you.

Step Four: Continue to hold your earlobes as you press your tongue to the roof of your mouth close behind your top front teeth.

Step Five: Still holding your earlobes and with your tongue still to the roof of your mouth, inhale through your nose as you slowly squat down to the ground as far as you can comfortably go. Keep your back as vertical as possible.

Step Six: Still holding your earlobes and with your tongue still to the roof of your mouth, hold your breath.

Step Seven: Still holding your earlobes and with your tongue still to the roof of your mouth, begin to exhale as you slowly return to a standing position.

Repeat this action six more times if you are able. You might not notice a change immediately, but after a few weeks, an improvement in concentration should become apparent. Gradually work up to 21 squats per day, adding one squat every three to five days depending on your stamina. Remember, go easy. Stay safe.

Starting the day with a simple, but powerful exercise like this could have amazing results on your physical, mental, emotional, and spiritual health. The crossover holding of the earlobes uses acupressure and energy flows to enhance the brain's function. This exercise increases alpha brain wave production. The breathing and movement improves energy flow through and around the body and increases breath and stamina.

Smoking and quitting

Smoking and tobacco use have been with mankind for thousands of years. In today's world, many people start smoking in their youth and get very addicted and continue to smoke their whole lives. Most people want to stop and have tried to quit many times.

I smoked a pipe and cigars, and I chewed tobacco for many years. Knowing that it was unhealthy was not strong enough motivation to stop. I tried many things to help me quit, such as pills, patches, gum, acupuncture, and others. Many of you know exactly what I am talking about. It is embarrassing to be so addicted to something and not be able to stop it.

Tobacco use is a dual addiction: physical and psychological.

The physical addiction means the brain is actually dependent on the nicotine to help perform some body functions. When the nicotine is not present, fatigue, hunger, brain fog, irritability, and other situations begin to occur. As soon as nicotine hits the blood stream again, things get better.

We become physically dependent on that chemical to help us feel good. There is one study that shows that the deep drag on a cigarette will increase oxygen in the blood. Deep breathing—without inhaling smoke—will do the same. In other words, we can become dependent on the nicotine and the physical act of smoking.

The psychological addiction has to do with stress and anxiety control. Even though nicotine is a stimulant, it can have a calming effect on someone who is anxious, and it can give a momentary break from stressful activities. Tobacco is a grounding substance, so it makes people feel more level. Some people who feel scattered or have lack of focus can concentrate better when using nicotine. It can stimulate conversion of glycogen to glucose, bringing up blood sugar. So it often reduces appetite and feelings of hunger.

These "positive" benefits of tobacco use are part of the reason it is so hard to quit. However, when you are ready and serious about quitting, there is a program that works well.

Start by mentally preparing. Set a date, your target date (T-day). Then, for thirty days, take homeopathic Caladium Seguinum 30C, one pellet twice per day. In addition, listen to some relaxation/stress control CDs.

On T-day, attend a live hypnosis session or listen to a hypnosis CD. Because the CD version is not as strong as a live hypnosis session, you might need to listen to the CD daily for the two weeks prior to T-day.

On T-day, stop the Caladium and begin homeopathic Lobelia 6C if you experience any urges. With hypnosis, some people do not experience any urges, but some do. Lobelia is made from Indian tobacco, which takes away the smoking urges. It basically tricks the body into thinking tobacco is present. Dissolve one pellet in your mouth every time you get an urge to smoke or chew. The urge might be gone for only 15 minutes or up to two hours. Regardless, just keep using it.

Your physical withdrawal should be complete after five or six days. And you are on your way from there to totally recover from the effects of tobacco.

Alcohol

Alcohol is another foreign, toxic substance we use to self-medicate, usually for stress relief. Science has shown that one alcohol drink per day can be beneficial by reducing LDL cholesterol in some Apo E genotypes, although two or more drinks raise LDL cholesterol. For some genotypes, alcohol is very toxic and should be avoided altogether.

Long term over-use of alcohol will gradually destroy the liver, leading to serious medical problems. Short term, we often use alcohol in social situations to reduce inhibitions, create euphoria, increase laughter, and help some of us men dance. Unfortunately, intoxication can lead to loss of driving privileges and is a factor in many crimes of violence and passion.

Alcohol use and abuse has been documented all the way back to prehistoric times. It almost always starts as an innocent self-medication, but soon leads to the trap of alcoholism. Most people who drink regularly need to supplement their bodies with vitamins and minerals because there can be extensive vitamin and mineral depletion.

There are ways you can stop or reduce alcohol use, if you choose. Beer drinkers often benefit from using herbal Hops. Hard liquor drinkers often find Kudzu / St. John's Wort by Nature's Sunshine Products (NSP) to be very helpful. Using a liver cleanse every four to six months will help protect the liver. We like either Liver Cleanse Formula or LIV-J by NSP as our liver cleanse of choice.

There are two homeopathic medicines that can help with alcohol abuse. The first is homeopathic Avena Sativa 3C or 6C, which has also been helpful for any type of alcohol or narcotic addiction. Taking one pellet once or twice per day reduces the desire for alcohol or other addictive substances. Two pellets can be added to the bottle of liquor or mixed drink to gradually reduce the urge to drink.

Case Study: LH was drinking 1½ fifths of whiskey per day. He called me one day and said, "I have to stop drinking, but don't know how." He had no money or insurance. He could not go to an expensive rehabilitation place. I suggested Avena Sativa 3C one pellet, dissolved in the mouth, once per day. About six or seven weeks later, he called again, laughing. He said, "It is 2:30 in the afternoon and I forgot to drink." He has now been sober for more than two years with no withdrawal symptoms or delirium tremens (DTs). He just forgot to drink.

Case Study: RI was drinking every night until he passed out. His wife of 40 years was disgusted with this and was ready to leave him. She put two pellets in his gin bottle whenever he opened a new one. After about a month, he slowed down to one drink after work and made comments like, "I am getting too old for all that drinking." Eventually he quit completely.

The moral or ethical question of giving someone a medicine without their knowledge is a personal one that you must ask yourself if you are in this situation. With the homeopathy, you can do no harm. Either nothing happens or the user will reduce their dependence on the drug or alcohol.

However, while secretly giving homeopathic Avena Sativa is safe; never give someone Antabuse, which is a prescription medication that causes vomiting if taken prior to drinking alcohol, without their knowledge. That could be very dangerous.

The second treatment for alcohol excesses is homeopathic Nux Vomica

12C, which is also used for a hang-over. I don't know if this will work for everyone, but taken daily over time, it usually reduces the desire to drink.

Strong support and tough love are also keys to successful treatment of alcohol abuse. Every person I know who has been successful in recovery from this disease has been involved to some extent with Alcoholics Anonymous (AA). All significant others should join Al-Anon, the AA support group for families of alcoholics.

I am not sure that a lifetime of AA is necessary. Repeating the words, "I am powerless over alcohol," tends to reduce ones self-esteem. Rather, we need to take control of our lives and take responsibility for everything we have created, including a craving for alcohol. I do think that, for many people, AA is a great starting place that provides some tools and support to break this difficult habit.

Anyone who needs daily support can register to receive a daily email of positive thoughts to help walk the road to recovery and elimination of alcoholism. See my contact information in the Appendix.

Mental Obstacles to Recovery

The mental obstacles to recovery mostly involve the activities of our mind that interfere with our ability to return to perfect health after any physical or emotional life event.

Walking on fire

As I stood by a bed of hot coals, I asked myself, "What in the hell am I doing!? Why would a seemly rational adult intentionally walk across a bed of hot coals?"

A few years ago, I had the opportunity to attend a Fire Walk. This was part of a personal enrichment weekend and the purpose was to face fear and do something that seemed impossible. This was to help me and the others there face problem areas in our lives with confidence.

There were 22 people in our group. We started by setting fire to a 20-foot-long pile of seasoned red oak. After about two hours of watching the fire burn down to red hot coals, listening to our instructor, singing, drumming, and mentally preparing ourselves, we walked across this bed of hot coals.

The majority of people walked across this fire without burning their feet.

I had a small burn on the arch of my right foot. Several others did get some burns.

What an amazing experience! It should be emphasized that this should never be done on your own and should only be done in a controlled environment with a trained instructor. Fire walks have been done for thousands of years, mostly in the context of cleansing rituals and rites of passage for teenagers entering adulthood.

It is not necessary to face one's fear in this way. It can be done in many other ways. But at some point in our lives, most of us will have to face our old, outdated fears. We often try to deal with those fears in self-defeating ways like alcohol abuse, drugs, over-eating, gambling, and so on. These might give us temporary relief but will never solve the problem.

Case Study: I have one patient who was 150 pounds over her ideal weight. She used a variety of weight-control methods and eliminated over 100 pounds and she was looking very good. One day in the grocery store, a man started to talk to her and asked her to go out on a date. She freaked out. She had been raped twice in the past, and she viewed her weight and size as her protection against men. She went home and ate everything in sight and gained 60 pounds in two months. Her comment to me was, "I feel safe again." Those old fears kicked in her fight-or-flight response, causing her to return to her old, safe comfort zone but also deprived her of what might have been a wonderful, healing relationship or, at least, a healthier body even if the relationship didn't work. This is an example of how facing our outdated fears can make our present lives better.

Focus on health, not problems

For the last 50 years or so, traditional medicine has focused on health *problems*. Many times in the past, I have told my patients, "You seem healthy. Let me know if you have any problems." As a result of this old message from me and from allopathic practitioners in general, most patients are not educated in ways to stay healthy. Sure, we tell them to eat right, exercise, stop smoking, don't drink coffee and alcohol. All of this is good advice, however, we are beginning to focus more on what's healthy in our bodies and not just the problems.

And we are also beginning to understand eating too much food is a problem and that proper nutrition is the basic building block for good health.

What we eat and how much we eat determines what will happen in our bodies. I recommend you rent a video movie called *Supersize Me.* It is an amazing eye opener to what happens if we eat a lot of food that is high in carbohydrates. Most of us do not eat fast food three meals a day, as the main character in the movie did, but when you think about what you eat, you might be surprised at how similar your diet is to the presentation in that movie.

The standard medical advice might not be the most accurate. For many years, I coached people to eat low-fat diets. When they did, many ate more carbohydrates and many became diabetics. It turns out most people need good fats, most need lower carbohydrates, and some need lower protein rather than high protein, which makes your body acidic and increases inflammation. We are not all the same. I will discuss fats and carbohydrates later in this book.

It seems that most people eat much larger portions than they need. If you hold your palms together to make a small bowl, that much space is same as the size of your full stomach. And that should be the size of your total meal when you eat. If you eat more than that, you will not have enough enzymes to digest that large volume of food and it will begin to be stored rather than utilized for energy. If you eat more than that amount of food in any one meal, then program yourself to leave some food on your plate. Leaving even a little bit at the end of your meal will re-program that old "clean your plate!" voice that most of us carry forward from childhood.

We like to use a program described by Dr. Peter J. D'Adamo, ND, in his book, *Eat Right for Your Type.* For many people, this has been highly successful, and I will discuss it in more detail later in this book.

Often, we also use the Apo E Gene diet, which I mentioned earlier and will again later too. This is much more specific than D'Adamo's Blood Type diet. By using the Apo E Gene program, food selection and exercise can be matched to your genotype so your body will have a gene-supported environment. This creates ideal circumstances for a long and healthy life.

Learn to focus on your health, do not wait for problems to develop and then try to fix them.

Thinking outside the box

You might have heard this saying, "Think outside the box." What does it really mean?

This refers to the limits we place on ourselves. The phrase is thought to have originated with some experiments done with jumping fleas. These fleas could jump 15 to 20 inches. They were placed in a box with a glass ceiling about one foot high. After they were in the box for a while, they would no longer jump higher than 12 inches even when the lid was off.

Other experiments confirm the same concept. Some great northern pike were placed in a large aquarium. They were fed small fish and minnows. After a while, a plexi-glass partition was placed in the middle of the tank with all the pike on one side. There was a two inch gap at the bottom through which the small fish could come and go freely. The pike would smash into the glass trying to get to the little fish on the other side. After a few weeks, the pike stopped doing that. Then the partition was removed. The pike would not cross that line where the partition had been and would actually starve before venturing across that invisible boundary that held them back.

After I graduated from physician assistant school, we would annually receive a salary survey that told the average pay with the high and low ranges for physician assistants in Michigan. This created a box that, in effect, set limits on the maximum amount of money any of us PAs thought we should earn and created a sensation of inferiority among those earning at the bottom range, or below. To break out of that box, I used one of Dr. Robert Schuler's techniques called Nobody Has Money Problems, Just Idea Problems, which I describe in detail later.

We often create comfort zones around ourselves. We might also have had limits placed on us by parents, teachers, doctors, and other authority figures. As we get older, if we do not remove those limits, they will affect us for our whole lives.

Often when people are diagnosed with cancer, the shock and the fear associated with that diagnosis can put them in an invisible box. They assume they are going to die, and all their body's natural defenses begin to shut down, causing death to occur sooner than if the patients were to choose to not be limited by the diagnosis.

Case Study: I know a man whose weight fluctuated between 200 and 300 pounds at least six times in his life. When he would near 300 pounds, he would go on a diet and get down to around 200 pounds. Then he would feel like he could begin to eat more junk food again and balloon back up to 300 pounds.

This is a case in which a comfort zone might have been too large for the person's health. That is, he was comfortable—but not healthy—weighing 300 pounds. He did finally learn to narrow his comfort zone and has remained around 200 pounds for a few years now. At that weight, he is able to be more physically fit and expand his activities in other ways that he couldn't do when confined by a 300-pound body (box).

Case Study: Mrs. B. was told she would not live to be very old after she had a bad heart attack at age 49. I have cared for her for over 25 years. She is now 94 and going strong.

The point here is simply this: You control your own destiny. Do not give your power to someone else or something else.

I have seen truly amazing things happen when a person thinks outside the box. Do your own research. Do not always accept the expert's opinion. It is refreshing to think outside the box.

Change

We are like plants; we are either growing or dying. There is no stopping this process.

Life is filled with cycles, up and down. In physics, the term *entropy* means that everything moves toward maximum randomness or chaos. That is the natural course of events unless something holds things together and brings them back to order. Life is what creates the energy to put things back in order. If you never clean and organize your home, eventually it will be utter chaos. So beneficial human growth means thinking, organizing, and planning for the future. This is the creative process that brings things all back together when they have drifted apart.

Deep inside, we all know that we're changing. However, our ability to change is limited by our comfort zone. On every issue, we have a comfort zone. Some might like crowds, and some like to be alone. We have a comfort zone about body weight and the amount of tobacco and alcohol we use. To change, we must learn and accept something new about ourselves. Even a small step outside our comfort zone can change us, just a little.

Change occurs when we no longer want to live the way we have been living, when we want to learn to live in a different way. Once we begin to make changes, it becomes nonstop. We learn about ourselves, change a little, learn more about ourselves, change a little more, and so on. We might not understand the process, but we do know that each step of learning and changing makes life better.

"How long can we keep getting better?" we might ask. For as long as we want. As long as we keep learning to know more about ourselves, life can get better.

Change is about choices. Small, seemingly insignificant, moment-to-moment choices made over a period of time will add up to major changes.

The medical community, the news, the television, the government, our religions, and our schools have conditioned us to follow the rules. And the rules include this rule: Don't change! But this builds our comfort zones and keeps us stuck in boxes that get stronger with each day that go against our nature and continue to live with unhealthy norms. Natural health is about change and taking responsibility for ourselves. Putting our health into our own hands helps us learn to break out of our old, limiting comfort zones.

Case Study: Several years ago, SP came to my office for a consultation for natural treatments for pancreatic cancer. His allopathic doctor had told him that he had three months to live.

SP talked about selling his boat because he would not need it anymore. He also indicated that he really didn't want to do that because he enjoyed fishing so much. I suggested that if he really wanted to survive, he had to act like it—including keeping his boat.

He also said his regular doctor had stopped treating his high blood pressure and diabetes. As SP said, "In my doctor's mind, he's convinced I'm going to die soon. That's why he has stopped treating the blood pressure and diabetes as aggressively as before."

But this man had made a different choice. He told me that he was going to live and he wanted everyone else around him to treat him that way too. This was a great and courageous step, a leap of faith. And it greatly increased his chances of living longer than expected, maybe even to be an old man. He did not sell his boat and he asked his doctor to resume treatment of the high blood pressure and diabetes.

He fished a lot the next summer and enjoyed every minute of it. He lived six times longer than his doctor had predicted, passing over about 18 months later because he was ready to go.

Fortunately, most of us are not faced with such a huge task of changing our thinking. But some of us are. Either way, change always starts with the thoughts in our mind. We must have a desirable, worthwhile goal. We then must mentally visualize and imagine ourselves having done the new thing.

We must talk to ourselves. Begin by telling that little guy, that little small voice, inside us to accept the changes. When we begin to feel it, when we change the comfort zone in our mind, we can more easily move, physically and emotionally, into that scary area outside the box.

Create in your mind a short mental movie of someone shaking your hand. Mentally see him congratulating you for having completed your goal. Then respond by thanking that person and by feeling gratitude within yourself for achieving the task. Play this movie in your mind every night just before going to sleep. Then, all night, your subconscious mind will be working to bring your goal into reality.

So learn to change and grow personally, put energy into life to push the chaos back into a more organized, desirable situation.

Is it time to change?

A few years ago, Barb and I had the opportunity to see Bob Seger in concert. It was a great concert and an amazing performance by talented people. Rock music is no longer my favorite, but it induced great memories. I have also learned that when an opportunity presents itself, I need to follow because there are always lessons to be learned.

The lesson was in my observation of the crowd. The first thing I saw was the incredible amount of beer that was being consumed. This, of course, necessitated many trips to the amazingly crowded rest rooms and a general disruption of the audience as people were coming and going every two minutes to fill the tank and then empty it. I told one very drunken fellow who was drinking beer while using the urinal to "just pour the beer in the toilet and cut out the middle man." He was not amused.

The second observation was the deterioration of saneness as the consumption of beer increased. At first, everyone was having a great time, singing, clapping, and dancing. This changed to a kind of rowdiness and then to belligerence and then wanting to fight. Two young men had to be removed from the crowd. It is too bad that some people do not put limits on themselves, like one or two drinks. If they had limited themselves, then the young men, their wives or girlfriends, the people who had beer spilled on them, and those of us who were subjected to this incident could have enjoyed the music.

The third observation was the distractedness of the audience. A huge number of people were using their cell phones during the show to send text messages, check email, etc. While cell phones are a fabulous convenience for urgent matters, it also shows the general uneasiness of people. Many are afraid of feeling disconnected or out of the loop. Many are deeply unsatisfied and cannot stay focused on what is going on at this moment. Many often want something different or to be somewhere else. Again, our enjoyment of a night of entertainment would be better if we can stay focused on what is happening now.

My fourth lesson was thinking about the words used to describe people who are using too much alcohol: "smashed, trashed, in the toilet, out of control, wasted, hung over, disaster," and so on. I am reminded of the recent email someone sent me. It showed photos of the destructive power of tornados. This is what the inner workings of our bodies must look like after any kind of excess. Yes, those damaged homes, towns, and lives can be rebuilt, but things will never be exactly the same as before. Some will never recover. And so it is with parts of our bodies that are "trashed and wasted" during a night of so-called "FUN." They might never fully recover.

According to what we know about the Apo E Gene, some of us simply cannot tolerate the toxic effects of alcohol. So what can we do? We first must decide to change our habits, which, for many people, means taking a huge step out of their comfort zones.

Then we start to look for solutions to help us with that change. AA and Al Anon certainly have been a great help to many people. Prescription Antabuse can be a big deterrent for the impulsive drinker because it causes someone who drinks alcohol to be sick and vomit. Saner, safer medications are homeopathic Nux Vomica 30C, one pellet before going out to party and one in the morning for the hangover. Follow this with homeopathic Avena Sativa 3C once per day every day until you change. Both will gradually reduce your desire to drink.

Let me emphasize: There is nothing wrong with going out and having a lot of fun. But there are ways to have great fun and not destroy your body while doing it. If this message has caused you to stop and think, then pay attention to those thoughts in your mind. They might be telling you, "It is time to change."

The Hundredth Monkey phenomena

I am not sure if this story is really true. Maybe it is just a story, but it nicely illustrates a point.

A number of years ago some anthropologists were studying the habits of monkeys on some islands in the ocean off the shores of Japan. They found one particularly smart little fellow and taught it to wash its food before eating it. He learned to do this quite quickly.

Soon the other monkeys in his family also began to wash their food before eating it. Later, this behavior spread to other monkeys in the clan. About the time when one hundred monkeys were washing their food prior to eating it, suddenly all the monkeys on all the islands, some thousands of miles away, began to wash their food before eating it.

This surprising observation became known as the Hundredth Monkey phenomena and has been repeatedly observed. The theory is that when a critical mass of thought develops, it somehow is transmitted to all members of the species who have that type of brain.

This same phenomenon is true in humans as well. It is part of the reason we have trends in fashion, the economy, and politics.

When we understand this concept, it becomes very important for us to develop our positive thinking. In the last few years, the economic conditions in my state of Michigan have been less than favorable, but they are starting to turn around. New businesses are coming into our area. Companies are getting tax incentives to move to Michigan. I see lots of commercial building going on. Things are on the upswing. In order to keep this momentum going, it is important that we all keep our attitudes positive, looking forward to a great future.

Buy or rent the movie *The Secret,* which teaches about the law of attraction. This means that what we think about we attract to us. When we, as a group, think the same positive thoughts, we can bring about more positive changes.

Barb and I stopped watching the news and reading newspapers years ago. We still choose to be informed about what is going on in our community and world, but we no longer wish to be contaminated with dire news and drowned in advertising—especially ads from the pharmaceutical industry that tell us that we are sick.

Many years ago, my mother, being very opposed to television, refused to buy a TV set for our home, saying it was "the devil's tool." It was the spring of 1969, when she finally broke down, and my parents bought a little used black-and-white TV. We all became immediately addicted, spending every spare minute glued to the "boob tube." It is interesting that, 40 years later. I have to agree with Mom, but for somewhat different reasons.

National Public Radio (NPR) recently had a story that some 30 studies over the last three decades have shown that excessive "screen time" with television, video games, and computers is definitely detrimental to humans physically, mentally, emotionally, and spiritually.

Last year, I attended a seminar on adolescent health. One presenter showed that obese children under age 15 had an average screen time of 5.5 hours per day compared to normal weight kids with 1.5 hours of screen time per day.

Research indicates that there is an 80 percent chance that an overweight adolescent will become an obese adult. Much disease, lots of agony, and over 300,000 deaths can be attributed to obesity and weight issues in the United States every year. And the studies show that screen time is a major contributing factor.

Another serious issue is mental and emotional problems related to exposure to violent situations. While the average person will seldom or never experience a violent death, the current 18-year-old will have experienced, through television and movies, over 40,000 violent deaths. I believe that insomnia, night terrors, ADHD, depression, anxiety, and many more unhealthy emotional and physical conditions are related to these experiences with television.

There are certainly huge benefits from television and I think most of us are more educated today than we would be without it, but … at what expense on the other, detrimental side of the coin?

So maybe we should voluntarily shut the boob tube down sometimes, reduce the screen time, and switch to more wholesome programming. Barb and I stopped our television service and only watch a rented movie now and then. I am amazed at how much more I get done during my work day, how much more sleep I get at night, and how much better I feel all the time.

Yes, Mom, you were right … again.

Remember the hundred little monkeys. What gets downloaded into our minds affects the thoughts of others as well as ourselves. So, monitor your thoughts and be careful what you allow into your brain. Together, we all make a huge difference.

Strengthen your inner defenses

The magic bullets of modern medicine that sometimes seem miraculous might eventually reverse on themselves and cause us some problems. Antibiotics, which have saved many lives, are currently causing some problems because the unfriendly bacteria have developed much resistance to these miracle drugs. This means that the bacteria have mutated to the point that antibiotics no longer will kill them.

When you get ill, and if the illness is not life threatening, wait two or three days to see what will happen. Let your body mount its defenses. During this time, you can use natural and herbal remedies like Echinacea/Goldenseal, Immune Stimulator, Silver Shield, Airborne, and VSC, an herbal antiviral made by Nature's Sunshine Products. Homeopathic remedies stimulate your own healing mechanisms and you might not need antibiotics.

Another thing that is being pushed today is antiseptic soaps and lotions. These soaps and hand gels should not be used on a regular basis. They kill off the weaker bacteria and allow the stronger ones to survive. This, basically, is selective breeding that results in tougher strains of bacteria. These products also remove the good, healthy, normal bacteria that protect us. Because many of these products have an alcohol base, they remove the body's normal skin oils, reducing some of the skin's natural protective barrier. Regular hand washing with standard soap is much better and, in the long run, healthier. Occasional use of the anti-bacterial products when a family member is ill is acceptable. But constant use is asking for trouble.

Our immune system needs the challenge of microbes to remain strong and active. We might get sick because of bacteria and viruses but mostly because of susceptibility to get infections. Why do some family members always get sick and others never do? Our immune defense is built up by exposure to many bacteria and viruses. The more things we are exposed to and the more we fight them off, the less susceptibility we have. Every time you use an antibiotic without letting your body build some defense first, the weaker your system will become. An occasional illness or "infection" might actually be your body's method of programming its own defensive mechanism.

Case Study: Nearly 40 years ago, I was a brand new physician assistant in Lakeview, Michigan. I was in the local hospital one morning working on some charts when I got a call from the janitor, a happy fellow named Duane. He also drove the ambulance for the hospital back before the days of Emergency Medical Services. He had to make a run to pick up a teenager and her newborn baby and asked if I wanted to go along. Apparently, the girl was somewhat obese and did not know she was pregnant and had delivered her baby unexpectedly at home.

So I grabbed an obstetrics pack from the emergency room, and we headed out. We arrived at a small trailer and were taken to a small annex with a dirt floor in the back. There on the bed was a tiny baby with the umbilical cord and placenta still attached. The new mom was pacing the dirt floor in bare feet. Duane and I clipped and cut the cord and loaded the mom and baby into the ambulance and raced to town. In the ER, I examined both mom and baby. Both were healthy and well.

I thought to myself, "This child doesn't have a chance, being raised in that home with the dirt floor." Much to my surprise, at every checkup, she was healthy and well. Always dirty, but healthy. It was one of my first lessons in the terrain theory. There were many more to come.

Incidentally, this child is now a grown healthy adult with children of her own. Her children, raised in a clean home with wood floors, had many more health issues than she did.

We can learn to *treat ourselves naturally*. Just what does that mean? It means to get well the way nature intended. Let's use the example of fever. A fever is a natural part of our body's defense system. Most bacteria and viruses that invade our systems cannot live at a temperature over 100.5. So when you become ill, your inner healing mechanism sets up a fever to help kill off the invaders. Because a few children have had problems and seizures with high, high fevers, we have taught everyone to treat the fever immediately with Tylenol or Motrin. While those things might help us feel better, using them will extend the illness because it suppresses part of the natural healing mechanism.

Another example is a cold with a runny nose. Yes, I agree that having a runny nose is miserable. But nature intended it to run so the invading organisms can be shed out of our body. Yet, we are trained by our health care providers and television commercials to take decongestants, anti-histamines, and steroid nasal sprays to stop the drainage. We might feel somewhat better, but those products only prolong the illness.

Another example is a cough. The purpose of a cough is to remove bad bugs from our bronchial tubes. So often we want to suppress the cough. Again, we might feel a little better, but in the long run, the illness is extended or more damage is done to the bronchial lining, setting up chronic, more severe lung problems.

The better approach is to figure out what nature is trying to do and then support that process. If you have a cough, drink lots of water and eat garlic and onions to liquefy the mucous and get it out of there in a natural, healthy way. Drink lots of herbal teas and bone broth soups. If you have an illness with a fever, take some good hot baths with baking soda or Epsom salts in the water. The heat will kill more of the bad bugs, accelerating your recovery, because most of the human pathogens, that is, germs that can cause bad infections, cannot live over 100.5 degrees. Magnesium from the Epsom salts will be absorbed through your skin, replacing the magnesium you lost from sweating. Homeopathic remedies such as homeopathic Belladonna and homeopathic Ferrum Phosphoricum will move you through the fever quickly. If you have body aches, your body is telling you to rest and stay in bed for a day or so. Pay attention. Do that.

If we constantly try to micro-manage our body and artificially fix things through prescription pharmaceuticals, our immune system will become under-active and non-responsive to those opportunistic organisms that are everywhere about us. Listen to your body. When you are ill, learn to assist your inner defenses rather than suppress them.

Mind viruses

I recently was introduced to the idea of Viruses of the Mind by a book by Dr. Wayne Dyer, PhD, *Excuses Begone.* In this book, Dr. Dyer helps us understand that we are all infected with these "viruses" in our thinking. These viruses, like physical viruses, will invade our thinking, reproduce, and be propagated by us to others. Some of them are detrimental and some of them are beneficial.

This work is based on the science of memetics, a concept created by Richard Dawkins who wrote *The Selfish Gene* in 1976. Later, Richard Brody, co-founder of Microsoft, wrote *Virus of the Mind.* He used the word *meme* (rhymes with cream) to refer to these viruses of our minds. He compared them to computer viruses. The subconscious mind, like the computer, cannot judge if information is accurate or not. It just acts on the information that is downloaded into it.

Dr. Dyer asked people from all over the world to send to him memes or excuses for not accomplishing their goals. He got over 5,000 responses. In his book, he lists 18 that were the most common and he gives the re-program-ming affirmation that we can use to change this meme to one that is more effective for operating our minds and our lives.

I do recommend you read Dr. Dyers book. I will share those 18 memes (used with permission) with you now. Along with them are Dr. Dyer's affir-mations (italic type) that can change the meme so it will build your self-esteem. I have added my own version. You can either use one of these or make up your own. The important thing is to make changes in the old, outdated programs that operate the thought system in *your* mind.

Limiting memes

It will be too difficult.
Dyer: I have the ability to accomplish any task I set my mind to with comfort and ease.
Huttinga: I can do anything I choose to do by making small correct choices.

It is going to be risky.
Being myself involves no risks. It is my ultimate truth, and I live it fearlessly.
I can do this, but if it does not work, I will learn and go on to do something even greater.

It will take a long time.
I have infinite patience when it comes to fulfilling my destiny.
I will do whatever it takes for as long as it takes.

There will be family drama.
I would rather be loathed for who I am than for who I am not.
I have loving support from those who care.

I do not deserve it.
I am a Divine creation, a piece of God. Therefore, I cannot be undeserving.
I am. Because I exist, I deserve a wonderful life.

It is not my nature.
My essential nature is perfect and faultless. It is to this nature that I return.
I am learning to overcome any genetic conditions and old learned programming.

I cannot afford it.
I am connected to unlimited sources of abundance.
I have always had and always will have plenty. Therefore, I am thinking of ideas that will help me afford this.

No one will help me.
The right circumstances and the right people are already here and will show up on time.
There are always qualified people looking for opportunities. They will help me.

It has never been done before.
I will attract all that I desire, here and now.
I am creating something new and everyone loves it.

I am not strong enough.
I have access to unlimited assistance. My strength comes from my connection to my Source of being.
I am not my body. I have mental, emotional, and spiritual strength to accomplish any task I desire.

I am not smart enough.
I am a creation of the Divine mind. All is perfect and I am a genius in my own right.
I am wise and exercise perfect timing. Everything I touch turns to gold. I am lucky.

I am too old (or not old enough).
I am an infinite being. The age of my body has no bearing on what I do or who I am.
My age and experience guides me and I learn easily to create a new future quickly. My youth and enthusiasm is my greatest assets.

The rules will not let me.

I live my life according to divine rules.

I function well within the rules of society, making adjustments for my circumstances. There is always more than one way to do things.

It is too big.

I think only about what I can do now. By thinking small, I accomplish great things.

I think in manageable pieces to accomplish great things. I make small choices every day to reach my goal.

I do not have the energy.

I feel passionately about my life, and this passion fills me with excitement and energy.

I am filled with vital energy every day.

It is my personal family history.

I live in the present moment by being grateful for all my life experiences as a child.

I release all negative events of the past and live fully in this present time. For as long as I can remember, I am in control of my body and my life.

I am too busy.

As I unclutter my life, I free myself to answer the callings of the soul.

I easily find the time for the beneficial things in my life. I accomplish tasks quickly, easily, accurately, and efficiently.

I am too afraid.

I can accomplish anything I put my mind to because I know that I am never alone.

I release my past experiences and move forward with faith and enthusiasm, creating a new past that works better for me.

Some of these old, limiting memes might apply to you. There are many more. I hear them every day: "Money doesn't grow on trees, it's the economy, it's the Republicans, it's the Democrats, it's the bank, I am too fat, I am disabled, I am sick, I have cancer, I am going to die anyway, I am not beautiful, I have a learning disability, I have ADD, I am too short, my husband (wife) is an alcoholic, I am bored, I don't care, I was abused, my mother hated me, I came from a dysfunctional family, I did not finish school," and many more. For every one of these memes, I can show you a person who successfully overcame it and has moved on to a better life. The famous philosopher Socrates once said, "It is the nature of an entity that determines what it will do and what it can do." Remember, if any human being has done something, anyone else can learn to do that same thing—and more—also.

When you find a meme that applies to you, read the healing affirmation or create your own. Then every single time you hear the old meme in your mind or from your mouth, cancel it and plug in the new one. Within a short time, you will be thinking and responding in a different way and your life will be getting better.

Mind your own business

Some time ago, Barb and I taught a workshop called 21 Ways to Find Peace. This was based on the material produced by author Byron Katie. One of the things she teaches is that we need to mind our own business. Ms. Katie says that there are three kinds of business: Your Business, My Business, and God's Business.

God's Business has to do with the big things that we really cannot control or change. Things like the weather, earthquakes, hurricanes, etc. If we worry about them, we create acidity and inflammation in our own bodies. We can take some action and pray for the people involved, we can donate money, and we can even volunteer our time to relief efforts. But when we catch ourselves thinking and worrying about these big things, we need to stop for a minute and say to ourselves, "This is God's Business and He will take care of it." Then relax and let it go.

My Business is anything that directly affects me. I must pay attention to and take care of those things. They are my responsibility. Only I can fix them. For example, if I smoke and it is causing health issues, then I am the only one who can correct that situation. No nagging from friends and family will make that change. And God does not care. He will help if we ask correctly, but He will not interfere if we insist on continuing with detrimental behaviors. If I am behind in my property taxes, only I can fix that. If I do not, then someone else—the government—will step in and take care of it for me. I must take care of my own business.

Your Business is the stuff that only you are responsible for. If you don't take care of your yard, it is your business. If I am upset about that, that is my business. It is not my business to fix your lawn or try to make you fix it, but it is my business to look at myself and how I react. My anger can make me ill, but it does nothing to you or to your lawn. I should only give advice or express my opinion on your business if you ask. Otherwise, it is best if I stay out of your business.

Many of us have grown children and we still think it is our business to run their lives. Let up. After your children reach the age 16 or so, your responsibility is done. If they make what you perceive as "mistakes," then they have to be responsible for them. Let them be. Do not meddle. Love them, pray that they will find their way, and let them go on their merry—or not so merry—way. It is not right if we take away their lessons and their chances to learn from what they do.

We are all here to learn lessons. Most of us have to learn to "live and let live." We must take care of our own business and let everyone else take care of theirs. If we spend our time taking care of our own business, then we will be healthier and more at peace. Try it. Practice. Every time you find your mind in God's business or someone else's business, step back and let it go. You will begin to feel less anxiety and more peace in your mind and body. You will be healthier and happier.

Remember: Mind Your Own Business.

You are what you eat

Every part of our physical body comes from the earth. We are 60 to 80 percent water. The rest of the body is made up of physical elements and compounds that come from the ground we walk on and the air we breathe. Therefore, we should take care of the earth.

Our food comes from minerals, plants, and animals—not directly from a store. Plants combine water and minerals from the earth and energy from the sun to produce the plant itself. Plant parts, seeds, flowers, stems, fruit, roots, tubers, and sap have been used for food forever. Some animals eat plants, and then we eat the animals. That is the way of the food chain.

Our body can produce most of the components of our structural body, but some parts must come through our diet. These needed compounds are called "essential." Therefore, when we look at labels, we might see the names "essential vitamins, essential fatty acids, essential amino acids," and so forth. When you see that term, it means we cannot make that material in our body and we must have it in our food. If we do not, deficiency diseases like scurvy, which comes from lack of vitamin C, and hypothyroid goiter, which is lack of iodine, will develop. In the past, deficiency diseases were much more common. Today, we know more about these things and we can supplement our body with vitamins, minerals, and fortified foods.

One big issue we face is toxicity in our foods. Many food manufacturers use preservatives and additives to extend the shelf life of their product. Last week, I saw bread with a 19-day shelf life. That bread must be loaded with something powerful to mummify it like that. The FDA requires these chemicals and compounds be within a certain safety range. That, in itself, is very good. And if we had only one or two additives in our dietary intake each day, we would be fine. But many foods that we eat every day all carry the legally allowable level of toxin. These, then, become cumulative, and the net effect is that, each day, we take in an unusual amount—an overload—of toxic substances. Some of these we can deal with and remove through our normal channels of elimination in the bowel, kidney, skin, and lungs. Some of the toxins we cannot eliminate and then we sequester or hide them in body fat to keep them from harming more vital tissues. This is one reason some people have a problem eliminating unwanted pounds. Eventually these accumulations will cause damage to some of our bodily systems.

Our body is no different than anything else we build. The quality of the ingredients determines the quality of the final product. If you want a beautiful garden around your home, you will prepare the soil, buy nice shrubs and flowers, and eliminate weeds. We cannot expect a nice garden spot if we plant weeds and do not take care of the flowers. Likewise with our bodies, we must start with good pure raw material and do our best to cleanse out any toxins that do get in. That way, we have the best chance at a long, healthy, happy life. So do your best to eat organically grown food and avoid the toxins.

You eat what you are

It is fairly easy to understand that our body becomes what we eat. But to understand that "we eat what we are," we have to look at how we select food.

In ancient days, many times there was not much choice. We ate when food was available and there were frequent periods of starvation. Today, most of us have an abundance of choices. If we had no outside influences, we would choose food that we needed. Some parents are horrified because their child eats dirt, but that child might be deficient in minerals and is trying to get them by eating the sand.

Studies have shown that children will select healthy foods until they are "taught" to select foods by taste. Parental modeling and television advertising are the two big influences on how children select food. Children learn by watching their parents. Remember that saying? "What you *do* speaks so loudly, I cannot hear what you *say!*" So if children see their parents and other relatives—or people on TV—all the time consuming coffee, pop, sweets, alcohol, and prepackaged food, that is what they will learn to eat. I see children in my office who would rather have an apple than a piece of candy. Why? Parental influence!! These children are modeling the healthy choices of their parents.

I also know children whose favorite place to eat is McDonald's. Now, we know it is not because of the exquisite cuisine or atmosphere at McDonald's. They want a Happy Meal. Why? Highly successful advertising! The fast food industry is very good at marketing to children. They know that if the kids nag enough, the parents will take them to McDonald's—or whatever burger joint is offering the best prize that week.

The bottom line is: we select food based on our thinking. I often see a thin person in a cafeteria saying, "I can eat anything I want and never gain a pound." Then there is the person who says, "This dessert will make me gain 10 pounds." Both are right. What we say and how we think about food has a huge impact on our bodily systems. I often have heard patients who are struggling with their weight say things like, "I sometimes find myself eating without even realizing I am doing it and I am not even hungry." These are examples of how our automatic thoughts have an impact on our body, our weight, and our over-all health.

So, if our automatic thoughts influence our food selection, we need to look at who we are. If everything is good, there is no need to change. But if we have allergies, are overweight, have joint problems, experience asthma, or fight diabetes, maybe we need to change our thinking. Learn to eat consciously and decide purposefully what to eat and how much to eat. Stop just eating automatically.

Therapies like hypnosis can help change our automatic thought process, but thinking and choosing with awareness and purpose is really a better approach. It puts us in control and gives us a sense of mastery over ourselves. The more control we can have over these simple things, the better outcomes we can have in our whole lives.

At The Healing Center, we offer Virtual Gastric Band Hypnosis to help people learn to eat consciously and feel full faster. I will discuss this later in this book.

Dreams

Dreams are actually an important part of physical, mental, and spiritual health.

Everyone dreams five to six times every night. We might not be able to recall that many dreams, but they do happen.

Dreaming helps sort out conflicts that we are unable to resolve during our waking hours. Dreams are associated with alpha brain waves, which are the most rejuvenating part of sleep. People can improve their recall of dreams by keeping a journal at their bedside and writing down part of the dream as soon as they wake up. Practicing this will greatly enhance your recollection of your dreams.

Many dreams have meaning. Some dreams have been called *precognitive* because they will actually precede some event. Six times in my life I have had a dream of someone driving a hearse. In all but one case, the driver of the hearse passed away within one week of the dream. This was really frightening until I understood what it was all about.

Most of us do not know it, but we can participate in our dreams. If you have a dream in which someone is chasing you, turn around and chase him back. That dream will never recur again. If your children have bad dreams, teach them the technique of "Monster Control." Just tell them to point their finger at the scary thing, and it will shrink down so small they can hold it in their hand and play with it. This is a great tool for teaching ourselves to make "molehills out of mountains."

Nightmares can be eliminated in adults and children with night terrors by using homeopathic Aconite at bedtime. Use 30X potency for children and 30C potency for adults.

Stress

Stress is a fact of life. Our goal should not be to get rid of stress because that is practically impossible. Rather, our goal should be to learn how to reduce its harmful effects on our body.

The word stress comes from the engineering trade and refers to the amount of tension required to break something. Stress, in medical terms, will attack our weakest system. Due to our genetics or past injuries or abuses, we all have some body systems that are weaker than others. When we are overloaded by stress, the weakest systems fail. That is why some people express stress through ulcers, others through high blood pressure, and others through headaches.

The first step to dealing with stress is to admit that stress might be causing some problems. Then identify and fix the problems that you can fix—the things that are "your business." Next, learn to eat right and avoid foods that could be causing inflammation in your body. Supplement with vitamins and minerals for a while, if needed. Learn how to relax your body. That does not mean having a beer or a six pack after work. That means identifying the activities or practices that will relax your body and mind. These could be reading, exercise, prayer, meditation and relaxation, or simply lying down and listening to your breath.

It is my opinion that we all should learn how to meditate in any of its many forms. Meditation physically relaxes your body so all our body chemistry can be recharged much like during sleep. It mentally relaxes your mind so it can process information better. Through meditation, both the mind and the body are more ready to handle the stresses of modern life. Read books, listen to CDs, or attend a class to learn to relax your mind and body. There are many places to learn relaxation and meditation. Ask at your local health store or metaphysical book store.

Nobody has money problems, just idea problems

The economic situation in some states might not be exactly what we want it to be. However, on an individual basis, we can all do something about our own situations.

I once attended a seminar by Dr. Robert Schuler of the Crystal Cathedral. He made the statement, "Nobody has money problems, just idea problems," and he wrote a book with that title. He suggested we write "idea generators," a list of 100 things that we had done in the past for fun or for income. The first several were easy, but after 60 or 70 things it became rather difficult to come up with more and more items. When you are doing the list, do not judge the items as good or bad, just put down everything that comes to your mind, no matter how silly or unlikely they might seem.

The purpose of the long list is to stretch yourself and your creativity. When the list is done, put it away for two weeks. Then take it out and read it over. If any good ideas come to mind, then begin to act on them. If nothing good comes up, then put the list away for two more weeks. Then read it again. Keep doing this until some ideas begin to germinate. Often, the ideas will come to you when you are not thinking about the problem, such as while taking a shower, driving, or doing some other automatic task.

If you have economic problems, step back from them now and take another look. What can you do to generate more income? Try Dr. Schuler's idea generator.

I strongly recommend reading Dave Ramsey's book *Financial Peace*. In it, he gives ways to get out of debt and begin generating wealth, not just living week to week.

Financial stress causes some of the worst effects on our health. Fixing that will greatly improve your level of health.

Think and Grow Rich

If you have not read the book *Think and Grow Rich* by Napoleon Hill, perhaps you might consider doing so. He was commissioned by Andrew Carnegie, one of the super wealthy people of the early 1900s, to research why some people were very successful at creating wealth and others were not. The deal was this: Andrew Carnegie would not pay him for his time, but if he discovered the answer, he would be able to apply it and become financially independent. Mr. Hill spent 20 years researching, interviewing people, and writing his findings. He interviewed over 500 financially successful men and women and over 20,000 so-called failures to get the data for his book.

He wrote his conclusions in a huge book of 2,200 pages called *The Laws of Success in Sixteen Lessons,* which very few people read because it was too big. The upper elite class wanted the book banned. They did not want the common man to have access to the secrets of their wealth. Hill later spent a few years distilling the big book down into *Think and Grow Rich*, which caught on and has sold many millions of copies. It sparked the positive thinking and self-improvement movement that has been going on since the 1950s.

The conclusion is that success is not just about making money. You can reach any worthwhile goal— money, relationships, health, career, sports, retirement, etc.—by following these easy steps. Simply put, we become what we think about most of the time. This book could be the step-by-step guide that you have been seeking to find your way.

Things sometimes look a little bleak. The economy could be weak in your area of the country. We hear all the bad news every day. Gas prices are high. People begin to wonder if they are going to make it financially.

We often forget that our mind is the most powerful tool that we have and, the best part is, the use of it is free. Stop watching the news. It is too depressing. If something big happens, someone will tell you. Read *Think and Grow Rich* and other success-oriented self-help books. Program your mind with good, positive thoughts.

A book like *Think and Grow Rich* might be just what you need to guide your powerful mind to help you get beyond some tough times ahead.

Outwitting the Devil is another great book, also written by Napoleon Hill. Based on an imaginary interview with the devil, Hill gives us some very interesting insight into the social issues people faced then and we face now. Interestingly, Hill wrote this in 1938, but it wasn't published until 2011 because his wife would not let him publish it for fear of being shunned by their friends. Talk about being afraid of the devil.

Laughter: The best medicine

We remember how the *Reader's Digest* column "Laughter, the Best Medicine" makes us smile. That smile and that laughter truly are healing. Norman Cousins, in his book, *Anatomy of an Illness*, tells us how he was healed from a serious connective tissue disorder by laughing.

In the video documentary *The Secret*, a woman tells how she used laughter and humor to heal her own breast cancer in three months. In the book *Molecules of Emotion* by Candace Pert, several scientists explain exactly how this works. In the video *What the Bleep do We Know?*, there are very graphic images that give us some nice understanding of our body chemistry.

In its simplest form, laughter causes a release of chemical endorphins, which are related to morphine. One of these is almost 200 times stronger than morphine. The endorphins act as mood elevators, pain relievers, and stimulants to our natural surveillance system to identify and remove foreign cells.

By intentionally increasing laughter in our lives, we can profoundly improve our health. Dr. Bernie Siegel, MD, in his book *Love, Miracles, and Medicine*, tells numerous stories of how people changed the outcome of their serious health problem by focusing on fun and laughter.

Case Study: I used to care for a man, WS, with Down's syndrome. WS was always happy and smiling. He was in his early 40s, which is rare for this condition. What was interesting was the lack of physical aging in his appearance. Most 40-year-olds have a few gray hairs and a few wrinkles. WS had no wrinkles, no gray hair, and his skin was soft and clear. Why? No stress and a life filled with joy and laughter all the time.

So let's learn to smile more, to focus on fun and laughter. When you are sad, do your best to set it aside and read some comics or funny stories or watch a funny movie. Practice being happy and enjoy a fun-filled life. It is a choice.

People who I work with often comment that I whistle while I am completing patient charts. I am occasionally asked, "Why do you whistle?" I used to say, "I whistle because I am happy." I now know that I am happy because I whistle. The act of whistling produces chemicals in my body that make me feel happiness.

Mermaid or a whale?

Recently, in a large city in France, a poster featuring a young, thin, tanned woman appeared in the window of a fitness center. It said, "This summer, do you want to be a mermaid or a whale?"

A middle-aged woman, whose physical characteristics did not match those of the woman on the poster, responded publicly to the question.

To Whom It May Concern:

Whales are always surrounded by friends (dolphins, sea lions, curious humans). They have an active love life, get pregnant and have adorable baby whales. They have a wonderful time with dolphins stuffing themselves with shrimp.

They play and swim in the seas, seeing wonderful places like Patagonia, the Bering Sea, and the coral reefs of Polynesia and Hawaii. Whales are wonderful singers and have even recorded CDs. They are incredible creatures and virtually have no predators other than humans. They are loved, protected and admired by almost everyone in the world.

Mermaids don't exist. If they did exist, they would be lining up outside the offices of Argentinean psychoanalysts due to identity crisis. Fish or human? They don't have a love life because they kill men who get close to them. Therefore, they don't have kids either. Not to mention, who wants to get close to a girl who smells like a fish store?

The choice is perfectly clear to me: I want to be a whale.

P.S. We are in an age when media puts into our heads the idea that only skinny people are beautiful, but I prefer to enjoy an ice cream with my kids, a good dinner with a man who makes me shiver, and a piece of chocolate with my friends.

With time, we gain weight because we accumulate so much information and wisdom in our heads that when there is no more room, it distributes out to the rest of our bodies. So we aren't heavy, we are enormously cultured, educated and happy. Beginning today, when I look at my butt in the mirror I will think, "Good grief, look how smart I am!" I am comfortable with who I am and enjoy it.

This amusing article made me smile. It is so true. We are all conditioned that everyone needs to be "ideal" looking like the people on the covers of GQ and Playboy. Granted, people who are overweight do have more health and mobility issues, and our goal is to help by finding ways to overcome the excess weight if it is a health risk for the patient. But it is equally important to be happy with yourself and to accept your body the way it is and love that body because it is the only one you have. The stress of always trying to be something or someone who you are not is also damaging to your health.

Thanks to the unknown author of this piece, which came to me via the internet.

Emotional Obstacles to Recovery

The emotional obstacles to recovery involve how we handle current and past events in our lives. Do our current responses to events help us heal or impede our ability to totally recover to perfect health? Do our memories of past events trigger thoughts and physical changes in our body that improve our lives or do they reduce our ability to return to our constitutional level of health?

Respond or react?

Here is the scene: I prescribe some medication to a highly sensitive person who is seriously ill. Will that person respond or react? Will the medication enter the person's body and help her recover back to perfect health (respond), or will it clash with the chemistry of this sensitive body and make the situation worse (react)? This is a common dilemma that some people must face.

Every time you eat something, your body asks this question but you might not even be aware that it is happening. Is your body responding so the food can be used as fuel for energy, or is it reacting and causing inflammation, mucus, pain, and other allergic reactions?

Respond or react? We are faced with situations every day. We make choices all the time. These situations are not necessarily good or bad. They simply are situations that happen in our lives. What we do with these situations is what labels it good or bad. Positive or negative. Do we respond or react?

If we interpret a situation as safe, we will usually respond in a calm, cool, resourceful manner. None of the stressful fight-or-flight reaction occurs.

If the situation appears threatening, we often react automatically, based on our prior programming. Most of the time, unless we have trained ourselves to respond in a positive way, our reactions are fight-or-flight reactions that produce acidity, high blood pressure, rapid heart rate, high blood sugar, high cholesterol, and many other chemical reactions that are harmful to our bodies.

How we respond or react is so automatic that we usually do not even think about it as it is happening. It is clear, then, that we will want to respond rather than react. So, in every situation in our lives, we must learn to sit back and observe what happens and check how we feel about the event. If we feel good, it means we have responded in a positive way, everything is beneficial to us, and we are increasing the quality of our lives and the quantity of our years. When we feel bad, sad, depressed, angry, irritated, worried, in pain, sick or other negative emotions or physical symptoms, it means we have experienced a fight-or-flight, stress reaction. These reactions will reduce the quality and the length of our lives.

There are many ways to slow ourselves down and learn to respond rather than react. But the first step is self-awareness. That means paying attention to what happens in our bodies and emotions in all situations. If we have a negative reaction, we can learn to correct it. If we respond positively, we can learn to make that response automatic. And soon we will have positive, healthy, happy responses to all situations.

To be happy all the time, learn to *respond*, rather than *react*.

Fixing the past

Our present life experience is the result of the influences of our past. The thoughts we think, the decisions we make today, and the actions we take are all based on our stored memories and the operating programs deeply imprinted in our subconscious minds. These past impressions come from what we have heard, what we have seen, and specific events that might have been either beneficial or traumatic.

This collection of past life events, stored in our subconscious mind, make up what are called *guardian filters*. If your life is the way you want it to be, wonderful, you do not need to change anything. However, if you would like things to be better, you can make changes to alter the guardian filters and, thus, the decisions you make and the actions you take. As a result, your life will become better.

To fix the effects of the past, make a timeline and list all events that need to be fixed. Below, I explain each of these is some detail:

- Grief, loss, broken attachment of any kind
- Lost love, real or imagined loss of a romantic relationship
- Abandonment, forsakenness, helplessness
- Humiliation, embarrassment, bullying, rape, abuse, guilt
- Fright
- The shock of bad news
- Worry, anticipation of bad things happening, performance anxiety
- Disappointment
- Burn out, over-exertion of the mind
- Anger, real or suppressed
- Homesickness, empty-nest syndrome
- Jealousy
- Dishonesty, theft, loss of integrity

To fix the above by altering your guardian filters, you can use these techniques:

- Emotional Release Letters
- Emotional Release Massage
- Meditation
- Mind Coaching using audio CDs
- Hypnotherapy
- Homeopathic remedies
- Bach Flower remedies
- Emotional Freedom Technique (EFT)

Each of the above remedies and techniques will be explained in detail in the following pages.

Emotional shocks that reduce our level of health

As you read this, get out the timeline of emotional events that might have affected your health. If you have not created that timeline yet, do it now. That is right. Go get some paper and a pen. Do it now. Construct a timeline of events and obstacles from the past that affect you in the present. The following will help jog your memory. We will use this information later on to heal the effects of these blocked negative emotions.

1. Grief, loss, broken attachment of any kind. This can be the death of family member or a favorite pet. It could be the loss of a job or missed opportunity.
    Case Study: I know a couple who built their own log home. They cut and peeled and cured and notched all the logs by hand themselves. It took over three years to build that house. A few months after completion, a faulty appliance started a fire and burned the home to the ground. Both have "never been well since."

2. Lost love, real or imagined loss of romantic relationship. This is somewhat like grief but subtly different. It has to do with loss of a romantic, sexual relationship, like when your "soul mate" dumps you. This loss can be real or imagined.
    Case Study: BJ was in love with a rock star in a band she had never seen perform. She had all his music and parapher-nalia. But she had never met the man in person. Yet when he married someone, she was crushed for months. She needed some counseling and homeopathic remedies to help her return to a normal life.

3. *Abandonment, forsakenness, helplessness.* These feelings arise from real or perceived abandonment. They can be related to a recent situation or to an event from childhood. A child might be "contami-nated" with abandonment issues if the parents were separated during the pregnancy and the separation happened four months after conception. This also applies to people who are homeless or

have no resources. And this definitely is a factor in the emotions of children of divorce with an absent parent. Some of us were emotionally abandoned by parents who were alcoholics or workaholics or simply ignored our requests for attention.

> **Case Study:** Starting early in life, AD heard his parents say he was a mistake, an unwanted baby, and if the birth control had not failed they would not have been burdened by him. Suffering from depression and anxiety in his mid-40s, AD was struggling and suicidal. This old programming was the source of his low self-esteem and self-loathing. We used hypnosis, meditation, mental house cleaning, and homeopathic Pulsatilla and Naturum Muraticum to help this man find his way back.

4. *Humiliation, embarrassment, bullying, rape, abuse, guilt.* The emotions that cause health problems in this category have to do with events in which we were very embarrassed or humiliated. Rape can fit into this group. Someone with a birth defect who was picked on and teased is often affected their whole life by these kinds of events.

> **Case Study:** I worked with a man who had suffered from a humiliation from the past. In the fourth grade, while standing in front of class reading a book report, he wet his pants. Now, in his 40s, he was still thinking about this and it was still negatively affecting him every day. Instead of allowing it to fade into the forgotten past, his subconscious mind had magnified this problem into something bigger than it was. With a technique called *revision* and a homeopathic remedy, he is doing very well, hardly ever thinking about that traumatic event from the past.

5. *Fright.* No matter what our age, we can have frights. The effects of this usually gradually subside. However, sometimes they continue to cause problems.

> **Case Study:** I once saw a little boy with stuttering problems. After taking a careful history, the story unfolded that the boy also had fear of bright lights and preferred to sleep

in total darkness. The cause of this was related to a visit to an emergency room after a fever seizure. When he regained consciousness after the seizure, the extremely bright lights shining in his eyes left him with a general anxiety and phobia reaction to bright lights. Homeopathic remedies resolved both the stuttering and the fear of bright lights.

6. **The shock of bad news.** What is the worst bad news you can think of? For some, it is the death of a family member. For others, it is the diagnosis of cancer or some other serious health problem. People tell me shock of bad news is like a physical punch in the stomach.

   Case Study: We saw a patient with terminal cancer of the pancreas. He did not have much pain, but he was very depressed and sad. The homeopathic remedy Gelsemium made from the yellow jasmine plant took away his shock from the bad news. In one week, he was totally different mentally and emotionally. He did pass away in a few months, but during those remaining days, he had much more peace and serenity than before.

7. **Worry, anticipation of bad things happening, performance anxiety.** Some people have a mental habit of finding the worst in a situation, always focusing on the worst possible outcome. A minister at one of the churches I attended a few years back gave this good advice: "Pray the solution, not the problem." Thinking of what we do not want, for a short time, helps us clarify what we really, really desire. Then we can consciously take our mind off the bad and play mental simulations of what we would rather have instead. Soon, we will create a new habit of looking for the best possible outcome.

   Case Study: DP was afraid to fly. His wife had booked an anniversary cruise for them from Vancouver to Alaska. The problem was the flight to Washington to get to the cruise ship. It would be a long way to drive and his wife told him that she was going with or without him. He tried a desen-sitizing program and even forced himself to fly in some small planes to try to get over it. Using the Bach Flower remedy Mimmulus every time when he had anxiety thinking about the flight and just before and during the actual flight totally changed his reaction. They had a wonderful second honeymoon.

8. *Disappointment.* This can be a subtle emotion and is often cumulative from years of disappointment by a parent. The child who is promised a trip to the ball park or the zoo and then cannot go due to the parent's other obligations will often lose trust in parents, other authority figures, and spouses. Other disappointments, such as not winning a contest, losing a role in a play, not getting into a particular school, or missing an opportunity, are often devastating. This lack of trust and sense of not being able to count on anyone can easily be restored by homeopathic remedies.

9. *Burn-out, over-exertion of the mind.* Many children and adults suffer from this emotional situation. Often these people are diagnosed with ADHD or hyperactivity disorder.

    Case Study: JF had severe insomnia caused by adrenal fatigue from stress and overstimulation from using caffeine to stay alert during the day. In addition to being highly sensitive to many foods and chemicals, she was stressed by her habit of trying to fix everyone and everything. (Remember to focus on your business and let God and your neighbors handle their own affairs.)

    She mentally trained herself to take her mind off everyone but herself and her own family. We suggested adrenal support, essential oil Frankincense, and homeopathic Arsenicum 30C once per day at bedtime. She eliminated wheat and dairy from her diet. At this writing she is much improved.

10. *Anger, real or suppressed.* It is important to understand that anger, as an emotion, is normal and actually a good ventilating tool. The trouble comes when the anger stays for a long time or when it leads to violent actions. Some families use the Five Minute Rule. This is very simple. It is ok to be angry, but it can only last for five minutes.

After that, it is time to forgive and forget. Holding anger releases some acidic chemicals into our blood that are very damaging to our tissues. This greatly accelerates aging.

11. ***Homesickness, empty-nest syndrome.*** Some of us do not realize the devastating affect this can have on some people. Sometimes when children leave home, there is a period of homesickness. Usually, a child begins to enjoy the new change in life and gets over this within a few weeks or months. Often, a child experiences homesickness when uprooted from school and friends, for example, if the parents move to a different town for their work.

12. ***Jealousy.*** This is a huge emotional block that some people carry their whole lives. The negative impact it has on the body chemistry is subtle but powerful, bringing about years of unhappiness. Often, over time, this emotion becomes chronic. It will eventually attack a person's genetically weak system, ultimately leading to the development of some illness.

13. ***Dishonesty, theft, loss of integrity.*** Most people have some event from the past that involves taking something that was not theirs. This can lead to low-lying guilt, shame, or embarrassment. We need to make restitution if possible, then forgive ourselves and move on.

The above is a brief list of emotional events that might lock us into some old patterns and behaviors that are not healthy.

Now that you have constructed your timeline of emotional events, think about infections, injuries, and illnesses from which you have never fully recovered. Add any of these physical traumas that still affect you.

First, do the mental/emotional work to begin to clear these events from you. Next, find the homeopathic remedies that most fit your situation and begin taking them. The dosage instructions for using homeopathic remedies can be found later in this book. For some situations, it might be best to find a professional homeopathic practitioner in your area who can mentor you.

I'm well aware that some of you will read this with interest and ignore it. Some will say, "Baloney." And some will actually follow my advice and write a timeline of events that have negatively influenced your life. I hope you are among the latter group.

After you have written your timeline, put it away in a safe place. Over the next few pages, we will discuss in detail some of the techniques mentioned above that you can use to remove the impressions of those past events that are still affecting your present life. As you read, take out your timeline and see if any of these techniques can be used for changing the effects of the traumatic events in your life.

Protocol for emotional release

Many times we have unhealthy emotional attachments to people, things, or situations from our past. If we hold on to these emotions, we cannot progress. We stop growing ourselves and get stuck in the past.

Here is the protocol for releasing ourselves from these emotions:

Using a pencil, not typing or using a computer, write letters to anyone with whom you have had any conflicts. Usually these are parents, bosses, spouses, ex-spouses, children, someone who abused or hurt you, someone you might have hurt, old friends, anything or anyone who has bothered you in any way even yourself or a diseased part of yourself. You are not going to send this letter. This process is for you and you alone. Chances are good that the other person involved in your past event has long forgotten it.

At the end of the letter, if it feels right, you may add the following statement: "I will no longer carry this debt for you Physically, Mentally, Emotionally, or Spiritually."

Then add: "I love you. I bless you. I release you. And I forgive you for everything I think you have done to me."

Author's Note: Write these endings exactly as they are written here. Often our recollection of the traumatic event has been greatly magnified from the original event itself. This is why we want to forgive the person for "what we *think* they did to us."

Read this letter and the ending(s) out loud three times and then burn it. You will feel internal emotional shifts, subtly or dramatically, within three days.

Write as many letters as you wish until you feel you have released all the old past baggage you have been carrying around.

Some time ago, Barb's email was not working correctly. I found that she had over 4,000 undeleted emails in her inbox. Our brain has many unnecessary files in it. Use this protocol as a delete button.

Because our personal development is cyclic, it is good to write more letters within a month or so. To see if there are still unfinished emotional attachments, simply think about the person or persons involved, or that certain part of your body, or that particular situation. If you still feel any unpleasant emotions in your head, chest or upper abdomen, then write another letter. Do this until all the negative emotions are gone. I once had to write a letter six times to completely clear it from my emotional body.

Every day, I hear people say, "I cannot change the past." While that is true, a memory of the past remains with us. We can learn to change how the past affects our present and our future. We can learn how to make our lives better and better. First, we need to know that we can change how we feel about the past. Second, we need some technology to help us do it. And third, we need to just do it.

If you have not yet constructed your timeline of emotional and physical trauma, sit down and do it now!

Emotional release massage

Associated with our physical body, we have an emotional body. Physical and emotional traumas store themselves in our body. From psychology, we learn that our physical body contains anchors or triggers that are associated with past actions or behaviors.

For example, let's say that your father was verbally abusive, and every time he yelled at you, he put his hand firmly on your right shoulder. Today 30 to 40 years later, if I put my hand on your shoulder in the same manner, that touch to your physical body will re-trigger all those past emotions. The triggers are stored everywhere in your body.

These things can be removed by an emotional release massage. During my second divorce, I was devastated. I began having pain in my upper back and shoulders and decided to get a massage. After the massage, I felt better, but the therapist said to me, "You know this is all emotional, right?" I said, "Yes, I know. I am working on it and I am meditating every day." She said, "You really need an emotional release massage." I had no idea what that was, but it felt right so I said, "Okay."

An emotional release massage involves applying certain essential oils in specific locations and lightly massaging these areas. When the therapist did this with me, I began to let go, crying deeply for what seemed like a half hour. She gently watched and let me release all the guilt, loss, anger, sadness, betrayal, and helplessness of that situation. At the end of the session, I felt cleansed. The next week, I returned and, this time, laughed through the entire session. The third time I had the emotional release, I slept through the entire session. That last session ended with a clear vision of my ex-wife drifting upward away from me disappearing into the clouds.

This important tool accelerated my grieving and healing greatly, and I am eternally grateful for people with those skills. Not all massage therapists do emotional release massages, so ask about their training before you have someone do this.

Meditation and relaxation

One of the tools we can learn to use to help us deal with the memories of past trauma is meditation. And 99 percent of us do not know how to relax other than to open another beer, sip wine, or mix a martini. Earlier, I spoke of relaxation and learning to meditate. It is my opinion that we all must learn to do some form of this. We must learn the art of slowing down, going inside, fixing the old outdated stuff, and creating new programs.

One of my mentors, Jose Silva, once said to me, "Your inner mind is like a football stadium with 26 gates. It does not matter how you get there as long as you use one of those gates and learn to get into the arena to see how the game of life is really played."

In the early 1980s, I was working in the plant medical department at one of the General Motors factories in Grand Rapids. The job was very stressful, causing me to develop an ulcer and high blood pressure.

I realized that I did not know how to relax. I did not know how to slow down my mind and let my body recharge and rejuvenate. Initially, a few beers after work helped me feel better, but that had other problems associated with it. So I attended a four-hour relaxation class. It turned out to be one of those life-changing experiences.

For the first time in years, I realized that the pressure I had in my chest was not normal. With the daily practice of the mental training exercises I had learned, my blood pressure returned to normal and the ulcer healed. The stress from that job was no longer impacting my health.

The results of this were so profound, I decided to explore further. I took another training program called The Silva Method of Mind Development and Stress Control. This was a four-day course targeted at teaching people to learn to use their own minds for the benefit of their own health.

During the class we learned to meditate. I had seen pictures of gurus with folded arms and legs, chanting in a blue haze of incense. So I had always viewed meditation as something strange and odd. In reality, meditation is very different than that. It is a way to relax the body and recharge all the chemicals that are constantly being used up while keeping the mind active and sharp. Having used this tool for over 30 years, I now understand what meditation is and what it can do for someone.

There are two general forms of meditation: Eastern and Western.

In the Eastern form of meditation, the focus is to get to a state of just *being*, an *awareness of being*, with no sensory inputs.

The Western version has three parts:

1. The Induction Phase helps us change quickly from an active, awake state of mind to a more passive, restful state of mind.
2. The Programming Phase involves mental pictures, which are much like daydreaming, and positive statements called affirmations. When we mentally see ourselves at an ideal place of relaxation, our brain thinks we are actually there and it begins to manufacture the chemicals associated with relaxation. Positive affirmations update our operating programs. Imagining something you have never seen before or visualizing something you have seen has a very powerful creative process associated with it.
3. The Ending Phase is a gradual return to an outer level of consciousness.

Daily practice of meditation will improve our lives physically, mentally, and spiritually.

Mind Coaching

Once I learned to use the mental training exercises, my high blood pressure and ulcers got better and I felt really good. This began a life-long quest to study how the mind can influence the body. Since then, I have studied many forms of relaxation, hypnosis, stress management, and alternative healing techniques.

For a few years, I worked with cancer patients doing something I called Cancer Therapy Coaching. Based on the work of Dr. O. Carl Simonton, MD, we used hypnosis, mental training exercises, guided imagery, revision, and prayer to improve the outcome of chemotherapy, reduce side effects, eliminate fear, and reduce pain. This was very successful but personally very time-consuming, and after a while I had to stop. I promised myself that someday I would record a CD that could be used for stress control, help with anxiety, improve physical healing, and assist cancer patients in all aspects of their therapy.

In 2008, the day arrived when I began to fulfill my promise to myself. I spent several months writing scripts for the introduction and five mental training exercises. Then I spent time in the recording studio to make the actual recordings. Finally, working with an artist, we packaged this in an attractive way.

There are two versions to this material. Some people, when they face life's challenges, feel reliance upon God. So we prepared *Christian Coaching for Perfect Health,* which makes reference to God and Jesus throughout the mental training exercises. Many other people do not share that view, so we also created *Coaching for Perfect Health* without the religious language. People use whichever version fits their needs. We believe there is no right or wrong in these matters, just different ways of doing things. I want all people to be able to benefit and both styles have had proven results.

I really want to emphasize the word "coaching." Most of the time, when someone has a serious illnesses, it is emotional human limitations that keep that person from accepting the perfect health he or she deserves. The person with the health issue has to do all the work to change his or her thinking to get a better outcome. But many times, the person does not know what to do or how to do it. Instead of years of study or trial and error, anyone can simply benefit from my experience to get the results they desire.

Therefore, *Coaching for Perfect Health* and *Christian Coaching for Perfect Health* were born. Later came two more CDs. *Pay Attention: Mind Coaching for Kids and Teens,* which helps children and teens to focus and concentrate. And then *Fit, Clean, and Sober: Mind Coaching for Recovery from Addictions* was created to help people change addictive behavior. My purpose is to not only help people become healthier, but to help them awaken to their own physical, mental, and spiritual power.

The CDs are available at: www.thehealingcenteroflakeview.com.

Case Study: JS had inoperable lung cancer, and she came to see me before she started chemotherapy. At first, she wanted just natural treatment. We have a very effective program in which we work with people on the physical, mental, emotional, and spiritual levels because cancer has roots in all of these areas and all must be addressed for successful outcomes.

I encouraged her to do the chemotherapy that the oncologist recommended. But we also worked with all those other areas. Hypnosis was one of the modalities we used. She was a Christian, so I had her imagine that Jesus was giving her the IV treatment. I had her visualize that as the golden fluid circulated through her body, it changed all the abnormal cells back to normal. She ended the program with imagining herself at 85 years of age, dancing and vacationing in her favorite place with her husband and family around her.

At her visit, JS stated that she did not want to lose her hair. I had her imagine, before every chemo treatment, that Jesus helped her wrap the roots of her hair in tiny plastic bags that would protect the roots from the poison of the chemotherapy. Amazingly, she did not lose any hair. She was ecstatic, but the oncologist was not. He used hair fall-out as a measuring stick to see if the treatment was working. This of course, frightened JS. So we backed off a bit. With the new program, about 25 percent of her hair came out—just enough to satisfy the doctor.

I lost track of JS a few years ago, so I do not know how she is doing today. But the last time I saw her, in 2011, she was 15 years post treatment and doing very well.

Hypnotherapy

As a teenager, I worked for a neighboring farmer. He smoked three packs of unfiltered Camel cigarettes a day. He called them "coffin nails," and, yes, that habit did eventually kill him. He had a book titled *Self-Hypnosis to Stop Smoking*. He never applied it, but I was intrigued, so I "stole" the book and read it. I practiced a few things, like a hypnotherapy technique on how to go to sleep quickly and easily. It was my introduction to that important topic, which I still find to be a very helpful tool today.

In general, hypnotherapy can be used to fix the past so the present and future are better.

Case Study: I have a patient who suffered from agoraphobia, which is a fear of public places, which caused her to experience severe anxiety whenever she was with strangers. She had not left her home in three years. We worked by phone or I made a few house calls. I used some of the Neuro Linguistic Programming (NLP) desensitizing techniques, but nothing really worked.

Finally, using prescription Xanax to numb her anxiety, her family loaded her into a car and took her to a psychologist/hypnotherapist I know in Detroit. He quickly determined the root cause of the problem. Her schizophrenic mother had caused her to become extremely sensitive. As a small child, she had to know what mood mother was going to be in before she came into the room. That way she could get a hug or hide to avoid a beating.

This ability to feel someone else's mood was a survival skill for this woman as a child, but the trait had grown so that, now, she could feel everyone else's feelings and hear in her head the thoughts of every person around her, even in public places. She was simply on sensory overload.

Using some hypnotherapy to deprogram this outdated survival tool, the therapist was able to teach her to control the sensory input, visions, voices, and feelings. Now, she can turn her sensitivity on and off as needed.

For many people, their experience with hypnosis comes from what they see on television, the movies, and stage shows—often used as a gimmick or a source of entertainment. But hypnosis is much more than that; it's a viable healing therapy. As a hypnotist, I simply guide people into a relaxed mental state in which the brain produces a lot of alpha brain waves. This state is what you feel when you daydream. In that state and with my guidance, the patient can remove old programs and install new, more updated mental thought patterns to think differently.

This is an amazing tool to help people stop smoking, change body shape and size, deal with anxiety, build confidence, and much more. I even helped an elderly lady remember how to play the guitar better. This is an amazing tool.

Another example of this tool is Virtual Gastric Band Hypnosis, created by Sheila Granger from England. This process helps the body and brain to think it has had gastric band surgery, which is placement of an inflatable band around the upper portion of the stomach to create a small pouch. This pouch is so small it will only accept a small portion of food. The patient feels full almost immediately, dramatically reducing portion sizes of meals and snacks. Both the hypnosis therapy and the surgery cause people to reduce the size of food portions they put on their plate without resorting to a diet. People eat what they want, but get full faster and select smaller portions without having to think about it. The advantage of the hypnosis, of course, is that it's not surgery and not physically invasive, therefore, there are no side effects or complications.

We present the Virtual Gastric Band Hypnosis program to individuals and groups once a week for four consecutive weeks. In our program, graduates may repeat at any time at no additional cost if they feel the need for some reinforcement.

It is important to understand that this in not surgery and it is not a diet. Participants just feel full faster and consequently eat less. Sheila Granger claims 90 percent effectiveness. I do not keep records, but we are seeing about 70 percent success. Several people have eliminated over 100 pounds in a year. Many have let go of 30 to 50 pounds.

This training is available in person individually or in groups and by phone. Go to www.sheilagranger.com/find-a-practitioner.html to find a practitioner in your area.

Homeopathic remedies

As you might have noticed, this aspect of natural health known as homeopathy resonates very strongly with me. As soon as I learned the basic concepts of this therapeutic system, I knew I needed to add it to my medical toolkit.

Homeopathic medicine is a system of therapeutics created by Dr. Samuel Hahnemann over 200 years ago. He was a physician. After his own daughter died of excessive bloodletting, he became very frustrated with the medical treatments of the time and quit practicing to work as a translator of medical texts and journals. With information he gained as a translator and his experience as a doctor, he developed a totally new system of therapeutics and spent 43 years working out the details.

Homeopathic medicine is based on the concept that "like cures like." It is based totally on symptoms and not on a diagnosis. Certain natural substances, if given to a healthy person, will cause that person to become ill with specific, repeatable symptoms. Hahnemann called this technique "proving the remedy." But that substance, if given to a person who is ill with the same symptoms, will heal. For example, onions will make your nose run and your eyes burn. If you have those symptoms from allergies, Allium Cepa, a homeopathic product made from red onions, will help you feel better. Likewise, Syrup of Ipecac has been used to induce vomiting if poisons have been ingested, but homeopathic Ipecac works great to stop vomiting from any cause.

The exact mechanism of action of how homeopathy actually works is not known, but it has proven to work very well. For example, the influenza of 1918, which was bird flu, killed over 50 million people. Homeopathic remedies healed 80 percent of the people who contracted these flu symptoms while traditional medicine healed only about 20 percent. Of course, traditional medicine has come a long way since then, but homeopathy does work well and is a safe, successful treatment for the swine flu (H1N1) and bird flu (H5N1). I'll relate more about swine flu and bird flu in coming pages.

Homeopathy is very safe. You cannot have allergic reactions to homeopathic remedies because of how they are prepared. You cannot overdose because homeopathy works on a vibrational frequency not the physical substance from which it is made. Homeopathic remedies can be safely taken with other medications, herbs, supplements, and oils. Just remember to have a clean mouth. That means nothing else in your mouth for a few minutes before and after you take the remedy.

Other than that, we don't really know how homeopathy works. But that's okay. We often use tools that we do not totally understand. Most people who use a cell phone or a digital camera do not know exactly how they work, but we still use them every day.

Many older people remember homeopathic Arnica. It is used for any injury, sprain, strain, bruise, or toothache. An ankle sprain, which would normally take four to six weeks to heal, will be better in one or two weeks. Every athlete and weekend warrior needs this.

Homeopathy can be used for acute and chronic health issues, and I find it to be a great compliment to traditional treatment. These remedies are nice because they can be used when no other treatment is available.

Case Study: Several years ago, TR came to the office because of her fear of the dark and loud noises like thunder, fireworks, popping balloons, and so forth. I treated her with homeopathic Phosphorus 30C one or two pellets every 20 to 30 minutes at the onset of thunderstorms or if balloons and fireworks were being used nearby.

After using this during two thunderstorms, she forgot to use it for the third one, proving to herself that the problem was gone. She later gave it to her pet Boxer who was also very frightened of storms and thunder. It worked well for him also.

So if you have a condition that arose from an emotional shock from the past, you might want to try homeopathy. Personal advice from a qualified homeopathic provider is always recommended.

Using the following list and reading more about homeopathy and its proven remedies, you might be able to find one that will help relieve the effects of past emotional or physical trauma. In a later section, I will discuss dosing of these powerful medications. I will also list a few Bach Flower remedies and will discuss those later as well.

Homeopathic Remedies for Emotional Shocks

- Grief, loss, broken attachment of any kind:
  Ignatia, Natrum Muraticum, Aurum Metalicum
- Lost Love, real or imagined loss of romantic relationship:
  Ignatia, Natrum Muraticum and Staphysagria
- Abandonment, forsakenness, helplessness:
  Aurum Metalicum, Natrum Muraticum, Pulsatilla, Aurum Muraticum Natronatum, Bach Flower Gorse, and Agrimony
- Humiliation, embarrassment, bullying, rape, abuse, guilt:
  Colocynthis, Staphysagria
- Fright:
  Aconite, Gelsemium, Ignatia, Staphysagria, Lycopodium
- The shock of bad news:
  Gelsemium, Ignatia, Natrum Muraticum
- Worry, anticipation of bad things happening, performance anxiety:
  Argentum Nitricum, Gelsemium
- Disappointment:
  Aurum Metalicum, Ignatia, Staphysagria, Lycopodium
- Burn-out, over-exertion of the mind:
  Aconite, Pulsatilla, Chamomilla, Coffea, Lachesis, Bach Flower Elm
- Anger, real or suppressed:
  Bryonia, Nux Vomica, Lachesis, Chamomilla
- Homesickness, empty-nest syndrome:
  Aurum Metalicum, Ignatia, Bryonia, Staphysagria
- Jealousy:
  Lachesis, Apis Mellifica, Nux Vomica
- Dishonesty, theft, loss of integrity:
  Natrum Muraticum, Staphysagria

Selection of Homeopathic Remedies

The selection of homeopathic remedies is based on the cause of the illness or on the symptoms generated by the body as a result of the illness. It is advisable to seek the advice of a qualified homeopath to assist you. See the directory at the National Center for Homeopathy. It will not list all homeopaths in the country, but will be a good starting place (www.nationalcenterforhomeopathy.org). The personnel at many health stores will know of homeopathic practitioners in your area. Many will advertise in the magazine Natural Awakenings, which is a national magazine with local offices.

First, let me give a brief explanation of how homeopathic remedies are prepared. I'll use the remedy Gelsemium as an example.

To prepare the remedy Gelsemium, the plant yellow jasmine is placed in alcohol for a period of time. This resulting mixture is called the mother tincture. This tincture is medicinal itself and can be given in drop doses to help relieve some conditions. To make it a homeopathic remedy, one part of the mother tincture is mixed with nine parts water or 99 parts water. The 1:10 mixture will become an X potency and the 1:100 mixture will become a C potency. The X stands for Decimal and the C for Centesimal, using the language of the Roman numeral system. The mixture is then shaken or succussed about 20 times. When this mixing and shaking is done once, the remedy is called 1X or 1C, depending on whether it is diluted at a ratio of 1:10 or 1:100. If this diluting and succussion (shaking) is done six times, it becomes a 6X or a 6C, with the X and the C depicting the dilution ratio. If it is done 30 times, we call it a 30X or 30C, again with the X and the C depicting the dilution ratio. And so it goes for remedies that have been diluted and succussed to whatever potency is needed.

The interesting thing is that the more the remedy is diluted and shaken, the stronger it gets. This does not make logical sense, but that is how it works. Exactly why, we do not know, but likely it has to do with resonance and molecular structure of water. Because of the polarity of water molecules, most likely digital imprinting occurs. It might be similar to digital code of computer language.

One of my teachers said, "If you take two homeopathic remedies at one time, it would be like having two choir directors, each giving different instructions." Therefore, even though some remedies are complimentary, it is still best to only have one remedy in your mouth at the same time.

Homeopathic remedies can be used to treat four kinds of illnesses: acute, chronic, intercurrent, and constitutional.

Acute illnesses have a sudden onset of a self-limiting illness or injury, such as an ankle sprain or a bladder infection and usually involve first-aid treatment.

Chronic illnesses have an ongoing set of symptoms that are not likely to resolve on their own. These should be treated until symptoms of the condition are completely resolved and treatment should be resumed with the same remedy if a relapse occurs. Most people have multiple chronic conditions that will likely appear in "layers." The layers are caused by successive events of emotional or physical trauma, like the events you wrote about on your timeline. Each layer is treated individually and usually in reverse order to the sequence they occurred. A layer is completed when symptoms for that layer subside. Then treatment can begin on the next priority layer.

Constitutional illnesses are conditions present from birth and could have a genetic or a prenatal basis. Constitutional symptoms might remain after a person has dealt with chronic conditions and any intercurrent symptoms.

Intercurrent illnesses are acute conditions that come up during the treatment of chronic conditions. According to Hering's Principle, attributed to Constantine Hering, MD, who greatly advanced homeopathy in the 1800s, when using homeopathy, one might re-experience certain conditions and illnesses that one has had in the past. This has been called a "healing crisis" and actually is part of the overall healing process.

Case Study: Several years ago, I cared for a woman who was taking homeopathic Calcerea Carbonicum 6C for degenerative arthritis, and after ten days, she got symptoms of a urinary tract infection similar to ones that she had in the past. It could be infection or a result of the healing. I suggested that this patient get a urinalysis to see if there was infection. If there are no bugs or blood in the urine, the infection should be treated homeopathically and not with antibiotics.

I also knew that she should stop taking chronic remedies while treating the intercurrent illness with homeopathic remedies for that condition. So I knew she would need homeopathic Cantharis to stop the sensation of burning that occurred with urination. Once the symptoms of the urinary tract infection stopped, then she restarted the original remedy for the chronic condition.

Homeopathic remedy dosages are determined by the illness, how long it has been going on, and by the sensitivity of the person with the illness. As a general rule, *acute illnesses* are treated with 30C and 200C remedies. Medicinal aggravations can occur when a highly sensitive person is given a remedy that is too strong, and the symptoms might actually get worse until the remedy is discontinued. Aggravations rarely occur during treatment for acute illnesses using these medium doses. If you are a highly sensitive person, it is best to take low doses at first and consult a competent homeopath in your area.

Case Study: I saw a patient who was highly sensitive. She had had eczema for years, which had been treated with all kinds of natural and prescription medication. When I saw her, she had a small rash on her wrist that she controlled with a little vitamin E cream. She wanted it to be gone. Being quite inexperienced in homeopathy at that time, I suggested a single dose of Sulphur 200C. In 24 hours, she had a horrible aggravation that broke out over her entire body. We used a variety of remedies over a course of two weeks. Finally it resolved, and has not returned in eight years.

I felt very bad about this, but felt better when my teacher, during my advanced training, told me of a case in which he did exactly the same thing.

The treatment of *chronic conditions* starts with 6C once per day and may be gradually increased up to three times per day if no improvement occurs. If there is still no change at three times per day, increase the dose to 12C, gradually working up to three times per day and finally up to 30C if needed. If no improvement happens at 30C three times per day, then we will retake the case and change to a new remedy, starting again at 6C once per day. It might take from three to six months to totally work through a chronic layer, but it is much better than having a bad aggravation.

Intercurrent remedies will usually need 30C or 200C repeatedly until the symptoms are better. Always stop the remedy for a chronic illness until the intercurrent symptoms have improved.

Constitutional illnesses are treated like chronic illnesses with small doses that are gradually increased to find the right dosage. Because these are conditions we were born with, length of treatment varies with each case.

When using homeopathy to correct old, suppressed conditions, begin with the guidelines for chronic conditions. It is highly advisable to enlist the advice of a qualified homeopath as you embark on this path. This can be done in person or by phone. You might want to visit our website, www.thehealingcenteroflakeview.com, then click Products, then Homeopathy to find a list of twelve common homeopathic remedies that we think everyone should use.

Bach Flower Remedies

Dr. Edward Bach (1886–1936) was a physician in England in the early 1900s. In 1930, at the age of 43, he became frustrated with traditional medicine, and he decided to search for a new and different healing technique. He spent the spring and summer discovering and preparing flower remedies. These remedies did not include any part of the plant but simply the dew from the flowers and leaves. Bach claimed that the dew contained the pattern of energy of the flower. Then, in the winter, he treated patients free of charge, keeping careful notes on his observations.

Rather than being based on medical research, using the scientific method, Bach's flower remedies were intuitively derived and based on his perceived energetic connections to the plants and what he perceived as the amazing healing properties of flowers.

If he felt a negative emotion, he would hold his hand over different plants, and if one alleviated the emotion, he would ascribe the power to heal that emotional problem to that plant. He would then research that conclusion with patients to see if he was correct.

He believed that early morning sunlight passing through dewdrops on flower petals transferred the healing power of the flower onto the water, so he would collect the dew drops from the plants. Later, he found that the amount of dew he could collect was not sufficient, so he would suspend the flowers in spring water and allow the sun's rays to pass through them.

Today, these remedies are made by placing plant parts (usually the flowers) in alcohol in sunlight for two weeks, then straining off the solids and using that tincture to make the remedies by diluting them with spring water.

Rather than recognizing the role of germ theory of disease, defective organs, genetics, sensitivity, and other known sources of disease, Bach thought of illness as the result of "a contradiction between the purposes of the soul and the personality's point of view." This internal war, according to Bach, leads to negative moods and energy blocking that causes "a lack of harmony" and leads to physical diseases.

Because his practices did not follow any scientific protocol and his methods were not well understood, they were never accepted by the established medical community. In his book *Heal Thyself,* Edward Bach wrote:

> "Disease will never be cured or eradicated by present materialistic methods, for the simple reason that disease in its origin is not material. … Disease is in essence the result of conflict between the Soul and Mind and will never be eradicated except by spiritual and mental effort."

Although the mechanism of their action is not well understood, the Bach Flower remedies are highly effective for mental and emotional difficulties like anxiety, depression, worry, mental chatter, and many more. They are safe and can be taken with any other medicine. They have no side effects. They either help with the problem or nothing happens.

These remedies will not fix an infected gallbladder, but they might help deal with the anger and bitterness that is one of the underlying causes of gallbladder disease, thereby fixing it long before it becomes a physical, pathologic disease.

If you have resentment, anger, jealousy, worry, hate, or other negative emotions, these Bach Flower remedies might be helpful. See our website for a complete list of the 38 remedies that Dr. Bach created, see www.thehealingcenteroflakeview.com.

Essential oils

Thousands of years ago, people used essential oils for medicinal purposes. We know this from the story in the Bible about the birth of baby Jesus and the three wise men who brought treasured gifts of frankincense and myrrh. The Bible also mentions the balm of Gilead. Incidentally, Young Living Essential Oils will be coming out with a new product, called The Balm of Gilead, in the very near future. The Egyptians and Chinese used these oils at least 6,000 years ago. Yet, today, many people are not aware that there are hundreds of essential oils available for our therapeutic use.

Pure essential oils can be taken internally, but most of the time they are applied externally or simply inhaled. The oils contain many compounds that can be identified, isolated, and studied.

There are two theories about how they work. First, these individual components of the oils have anti-inflammatory, anti-viral, anti-bacterial, and anti-cancer properties. When the oil is applied to the skin or inhaled, it is absorbed and circulated through the body. The active ingredients then "do their thing" within the body, adjusting the chemistry based on its individual properties.

The second theory has to do with resonant vibrational frequencies. Every subatomic particle, atom, molecule, cell, tissue, organ, and the body as a whole has a resonant vibrational frequency. The composite of these seven layers is an electromagnetic field and it is often called the *aura*. When there is disease within the body, changes in the resonant vibrational frequency in the aura also occur. The changes can be at any level. This is actually the basis for magnetic resonance imaging (MRI) with which many of us are familiar.

The oils have the ability to bring the abnormal frequency back to normal through the principle of harmonics. All musical instruments are based on these laws of physics. This simply means that one thing that is vibrating can cause something else to vibrate at the same rate or frequency. As far as the oils are concerned, research has determined which oils can influence which frequencies within our bodies. We can then educate ourselves to know which oils can be used to reduce pain and inflammation, which oils can remove bacteria and viruses, which oils can change the vibrational frequency of tumors and cancers, and so on. Understanding this, we realize essential oils represent a complete therapeutic system to help us improve our health.

I personally am not an expert in this field, but we use the reference material created by Dr. Gary Young, ND, pioneer and founder of Young Living Essential Oils, to select the proper oils for a particular condition. To my knowledge, these are the only essential oils that can safely be taken internally.

Here are a few examples of how some oils are used for emotional conditions.

Case Study: AS is a patient who is a high school student with anxiety about taking tests and fear of public speaking. While studying for a test, she uses an old blend called Brain Power and Focus. She also uses Valor and homeopathic Gelsemium 30C before taking tests. Because of school rules, she is required to go down to the school office to take them, but they reduce her anxiety and allow her to focus on her tests, improving her grades.

Case Study: TB is a young man with asthma and anxiety, two conditions that commonly go together because the fear of death when one cannot breathe is very strong. By eliminating foods that he was sensitive to, his asthma improved. In addition, we recommended two essential oils, Joy and White Angelica. Both have been highly beneficial for treatment of both anxiety and asthma. Depending on the situation, they can be inhaled or taken orally in a gel capsule diluted with two drops of olive oil on an as-needed basis.

Case Study: KS has a lot of depression. She lived in a house contaminated with mold for three years. It is my opinion that the mold is responsible for the brain chemistry imbalance that caused her depression symptoms. I treated her with an oil blend called Thieves, which is known for its anti-fungal properties. Internally taking two drops in a gel capsule diluted with two drops of olive oil twice a day for two months has made a lot of difference in her emotional state as well as her general energy. I honestly do not know the mechanism of this, but have seen it work in several other cases of depression in sensitive people with mold exposure.

Emotional Freedom Technique (EFT) or meridian tapping

The meridian system is the method by which energy flows through the body. Chinese medicine, acupuncture, and the martial arts use this energy flow system. There are no physical structures like nerves or arteries through which this energy flows, rather it is thought that this flow of energy might go through an elaborate network of water molecules that are bound together by their polar charges. This is yet to be proven, but it makes sense to me because this energy is related to auras, the energy field that flows through and around us, that I discussed earlier in relationship to the electromagnetic field around our body.

Far Eastern and East Indian cultures have believed for centuries that this energy flows in patterns into and out of centers located along the spine. These energy centers are also called *chakra*, a word that comes from Sanskrit and means vortex or whirlpool.

There are seven basic energy centers that, like a spinning vortex, project from the front and from the back of the body in seven locations along the spine.

- The first or root chakra projects downward from an area between the genitals and the rectum.
- The second comes from an area above the pubic bone.
- The third comes from the solar plexus area between the rib cage and the navel.
- The fourth, called the heart chakra, is found in the heart area.
- The fifth is in the throat and back of the neck.
- The sixth, in the center of the forehead, has been called "the third eye."
- And the seventh, called the crown chakra, projects straight up from the top of the head.

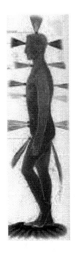

Drawing of the seven main Energy Centers

When our emotions get stuck, the flow in this meridian energy system is altered. When this happens, the spin of energy in the chakras and the flow in the body can change or reverse direction. Have you ever met someone who reverses everything you say or someone who opposes everything? This person probably has a reversal of energy flow, which we call "reverse polarity." A practitioner who does energy work can return that flow to normal.

Highly sensitive people can see and feel this energy. Kirlian photography has filmed it. Chiropractors feel it. Acupuncturists, Reiki masters, and hands-on healers manipulate it to help heal people.

In 2010 on the television series The Learning Channel (TLC), some of you might have seen Paul McKenna using tapping techniques to help people eliminate food cravings. Thought Field Therapy (TFT) created by Dr. Roger Callaghan is the foundation of all these tapping methods. They work by releasing stuck energy in the meridian system.

Barb and I discussed this with Dr. Gary Laundre, PhD, from Grand Rapids, Michigan, who wrote the book *The Happiness Code*. This book is based on Emotional Freedom Technique (EFT), which is the latest version of TFT. EFT can be applied by a therapist, or anyone can easily use it on themselves. The information in *The Happiness Code* is easy to use. For a great easy-to-understand article by Dr. Laundre on tapping techniques, see www. thehappinesscode.com/12345.pdf.

These techniques can be used to eliminate major fears and phobias, panic attacks, guilt, shame, embarrassment, anger, grief over lost love, anxiety and depression as well as addictive urges and obsessive behavior.

In the pineal gland and hypothalamus, which are located in the limbic area of our brain, we house something called *guardian filters*. This is not an actual physical structure but, rather, a mental mechanism that filters information between our conscious and subconscious mind. It is much like the spam filter and the firewalls in your computer. These filters are made up of a composite of our beliefs, past emotional traumas, past illnesses, genetic memory, and head injuries. If the information stored in the guardian filter is not accurate, we can react in an inappropriate manner.

Case Study: I have a patient who has a heights phobia caused by a mishap in childhood in which he nearly fell off a water tower. Now, 40 years later, he still feels the panic from simply watching a movie in which someone is looking over a cliff. He used meridian tapping every time he felt the panic in his chest. After doing the tapping eight or ten times, that feeling was no longer triggered by watching a movie. This disconnected the mental image from the release of the fight-or-flight chemicals that gave the panic feelings.

The misinterpretation in the filter is what causes us to have emotional reactions that do not fit the circumstance.

Spiritual Obstacles to Recovery

The spiritual obstacles to recovery involve the aspects of life that extend beyond the physical, mental, and emotional realms that we can see, hear, or touch. It is that invisible spiritual world where many of us have little experience. We need peace of mind in this area of our lives in order to have a long, peaceful, healthy life.

Religious or spiritual?

I have often heard people make the comment, "I am spiritual, not religious." To help explain this, let me share a story from Jose Silva. Once he asked us the question, "Why do you have the religion that you currently practice?" His answer was that, for most people, their religion was determined by where and to what parents they were born. He was born in Mexico. Since a high percentage of religious people in Mexico are Catholic, that is the religion he "inherited" and it was the religion he practiced until he passed over.

Silva was a radio repairman in the US military. After his military service was completed, he returned home and began an electronics repair business. He was an accomplished problem solver. So when he asked himself this question, "Why am I a Catholic?" he decided to study the foundation of all the major religions. His conclusion was that it really did not matter what religion a person identified with; the important thing was congruence. If someone professed to believe in something then, to be spiritually healthy, that person would need to practice that belief. We need to "walk our talk."

This concept made a great deal of sense to me. I recalled my childhood when I questioned some of my parents' beliefs. We grew up in a small protestant denomination of the Christian Reformed Church. We lived in the country. The nearest neighbor kids were from a Catholic family. My mom did not want us to play with them because, she said, "They were going to hell." The funny thing was that their parents were saying the same thing about us.

In 2005, I had an interesting experience. Barb and I were attending a class at a nearby bookstore. As we went around the room introducing ourselves, the woman sitting next to me introduced herself as a witch. I had a panic attack, nearly jumping out of my chair. I literally sat through much of the class with my hands under the table with my fingers held in the sign of the cross. When I got home, I realized that I knew nothing about witches or Wiccan and pagan religions. So I read some books, searched the web, and talked to two people who live in our community and practice these traditions. I found that witchcraft is not Satan worship, that witches do not practice animal or human sacrifices, or perform rituals that were the basis of any of my other fears. My panic was from lack of knowledge. Today, I still choose not to practice those beliefs, but I no longer fear them or their practitioners.

It has been my conclusion, after studying the major religions and many minor traditions, that they all have been created by humankind in an attempt to help explain our unseen spiritual dimension and our relationship with God. Our mind is the connecting link between the objective physical world of the body and the subjective invisible spiritual world. We must learn to use it wisely.

A daily spiritual practice is very important. How you do that is your choice. As I mentioned earlier, the spiritual dimension is like a football stadium with 26 gates. How we get inside is not as important as the fact that we go there and that we use that dimension for our spiritual evolution.

Barb and I have traveled a lot to many nations. We have seen and experienced the religious practices of many people of various major faith groups. They are all different, but have a similar thread. The similarity is their method of entering the spiritual world. For my parents, it was daily devotions with Bible reading and prayer. In Egypt, we heard the Islamic "call to pray" and saw Muslims kneel to pray five times each day. In China, mediation and tai chi were used to enter that dimension.

It is actually important for our health—physical, mental, emotional, and spiritual—to have beliefs and congruently practice them daily. The great thing is that you get to choose and whatever you decide is good.

Napoleon Hill talked about the master mind. This is a gathering of people who come together for a common purpose. The group size can be two or thousands. The master mind is the entity that develops that is greater than the sum of the individuals who make up the group. Churches are master minds. They give people great social contacts with people of similar thinking. This forms a comfort zone and a foundation for trust among members. This comfort zone can be beneficial if the congregation supports each other. Or it can be limiting if individuals never go outside that box.

There is no good or bad about all this; it is just what exists. How we judge faiths or faith practitioners is based on our guardian filters. These are what determine whether something is good or bad in our own eyes. I think that my filters are quite broad in scope. I believe we are social beings, religious beings, and spiritual beings.

This section of the book will discuss briefly some of my thoughts on this topic. It does not matter if you agree or disagree. My purpose is to stimulate thought, to expand your thinking, to add new points of reference for your brain, and to allow you to determine if you might want to modify your guardian filters. If things are working in your life, then you are living a life that is meaningful and correct for you. If you are experiencing physical, mental, or emotional issues—or *dis-ease*—then you might wish to re-evaluate your beliefs.

Pray the solution

I have already used this information in relation to why some of us get ill, but it is so important that I have chosen to share it again—in a new context.

Gregg Braden is a quantum physicist and a philosopher. Much of his work relates to his long search through the writings and sacred texts of ancient cultures for a more effective form of prayer. Gregg says that the classic method of many of our prayers, that is, asking God *for* what we want, actually cancels out our request. We often begin a prayer by acknowledging that we do not have what we want.

Remember Gregg's friend, David, who said, "I said that I would *pray rain*. If I have *prayed for rain*, it would never happen." Then Gregg asked, "If you didn't pray for rain, then what did you do?"

"It's simple," David replied. "I began to have the feeling of what rain feels like. I felt the feeling of rain on my body, and what it feels like to stand with my naked feet in the mud in our village plaza because there has been so much rain. I smelled the smells of rain on the earthen walls in our village, and felt what it feels like to walk through fields of corn chest high because there has been so much rain."

David had used his thoughts, feelings, and emotions to perceive what he desired as an already accomplished fact.

For many years, I have taught people to pray the solution, not the problem. This story from Gregg Braden illustrates how to do that. I thought it was worthwhile to pass along. We can learn to *pray health*, not for health or the removal of the disease.

Rev. Don Piper, in his book *Ninety Minutes in Heaven*, describes how he was prayed back to life by a fellow pastor 90 minutes after being pronounced dead after a serious motor vehicle accident. Here is a synopsis from the back cover of the book.

As he is driving home from a minister's conference, Baptist minister Don Piper collides with a semi-truck that crosses into his lane. He is pronounced dead at the scene. For the next 90 minutes, Piper experiences heaven where he is greeted by those who had influenced him spiritually. He hears beautiful music and feels true peace.

Back on earth, a passing minister who had also been at the conference is led to pray for Don even though he knows the man is dead. Piper miraculously comes back to life and the bliss of heaven is replaced by a long and painful recovery. For years, Piper kept his heavenly experience to himself. Finally, however, friends and family convinced him to share his remarkable story.

Interestingly, Piper uses exactly the same words as Gregg Braden's friend. He was "prayed back to life" by the passing minister. There is something here for all of us to pay attention to. The word "pray" is an action verb. It can be used to create an outcome. Learn to use it.

Energy medicine and the science of hands-on healing

Imagine the scene. A small Brazilian village in 2009. A line of people in a clean white-and-blue building called The Casa. A man named John of God has his hands on another man's head. After a few minutes, the "patient" stands up, shakes his head a little, smiles, thanks the man, and leaves. I watched this scene in amazement as the healer continued to work on people with all sorts of maladies.

John of God cut out a small cyst with a pocket knife. There was very little bleeding, no infection, and the incision was almost completely healed in less than 24 hours.

He placed one hand on the abdomen of a child with colic. He placed the other hand on the child's back. He closed his eyes, bowed his head, and vibrated his hands slightly. The child stopped crying immediately.

He scraped the cornea of another man with a paring knife as a treatment for cataracts. In most cases, the cataracts will dissolve in six months or so.

John of God told us, through an interpreter, "God provides the power; I just tell it where to go."

This seemed miraculous, but there is an explanation that makes sense.

Barb and I spent two weeks at The Casa. Although we did not have serious health issues, it was an amazing experience to stand before this healer, have "spiritual surgery," meditate for seven hours a day, and talk to some of the thousands of people who came to see John of God every week.

Scientists have studied this man. They found that he had a zone around his hands, extending about 14 inches, that could sterilize bacteria, viruses, and fungi that had been growing in Petri dishes. How is this possible? The theory is that we have electromagnetic fields around our body, especially around our hands. The composite of these layers of the electromagnetic fields are called the aura. These fields have been photographed using Kirlian photography techniques. We all have this aura. The Brazilian healer, John of God, had probably been born with a stronger than average flow of energy into his hands, it was never programmed out of him by parents or other authority figures, and he had learned to strengthen it as he used it to do his healing work.

We all have this energy to one degree or another. Many people are being trained to increase and use it. Reiki energy healing was created in Japan thousands of years ago. Ama-Deus energy healing comes from South America and is also thousands of years old. Jesus healed with his hands, and many Christians have used "laying on of hands" for healing. I know Amish people who can "hold pain" for someone who is ill and hurting. Quantum Healing, Touch for Health, and Therapeutic Massage are more modern systems that are effective energy healing methods.

The energy around our body is in seven layers, one layer each from the energy of all the subatomic particles, atoms, molecules, cells, tissues, organs, and finally the organism as a whole. When we meet someone, we often feel an attraction or repulsion. That's because we are feeling the energy fields around that person. The field can be a few inches thick or as large as 50 feet around a person. When a person is ill, changes in the fields can be detected by those who are sensitive to the energy. The energy healing technique uses the energy field of one person to correct the defects in the field of the ill person by harmonic vibrations.

This is what the Brazilian healer did and what anyone trained in these other techniques can do. The energy can *only* be transmitted, however, if the patient is willing to receive. There must be expectancy. We all have free will to accept or reject the effects of the energy of another person.

We can learn to use this energy to improve our health and that of our families. We suggest you explore some of these methods for yourself. Please do not discourage your children if they display some ability in this area. Many autistic children can do this.

Intuition and psychic phenomenon

When I was growing up, I remember Mom talking about dreams that came true and learning to pay attention to those little feelings that we sometimes get. At the time, I really did not pay too much attention to either the feelings or Mom's words.

But as I got older, I noticed many times that I would get a feeling in my chest that something was wrong. I usually could not tell what was wrong but later would find out that someone had been in an accident or something like that. Often when leaving the house, I would get a feeling that I was forgetting something. Like almost everyone, you have probably had the experience of thinking about someone and then they call you on the phone or you meet them on the street. You have likely noticed when you meet someone for the first time that you often get good or bad feelings about that person.

What is all that? It seems that we, as humans—as well as animals—can somehow communicate through something other than our five physical senses. We can get visions in our minds, voices in our heads, and feelings in our chest or gut. This is not understood very well, but the idea is that we get information about an event far enough in advance that we can fix it soon enough to ensure our survival.

All mothers have this sensation of protection for their young. They use it to know what their infant children need. Parents keep this connection for life.

Case Study: I once had a patient who had agoraphobia, which is fear of public places. She could hear other people's thoughts in her head as if they were talking to her out loud. So when she went to the store, she was overwhelmed with all that psychic noise. It was literally driving her crazy. With the help of some hypnotherapy, homeopathic Argentum Nitricum, and Bach Flower Elm, she learned how to control this and use it for her benefit. She now makes a living as a medical intuitive.

Remember, all of us have intuition whether we use it or not. Begin to pay attention to those little inner messages; you will be surprised at what happens.

Recently, Barb and I were on a cruise. Someone's guitar case, was mistakenly delivered to our room. When it was convenient, I went down to the front desk to report this. As I was describing this situation to the receptionist, the man standing next to me, overhearing our conversation, looked over and said, "That is my guitar case." He described it perfectly and came to my room to retrieve his belongings. The remarkable aspect of this story is that the owner didn't immediately report that the guitar case was missing, nor did I immediately report that I had found it. But both of us did show up at the receptionist's office at the same time. This type of synchronicity or coincidence will happen all the time when you begin to listen to your intuition.

The seer, the prophet, the medium, the psychic

Some time ago at The Healing Center, we sponsored a psychic fair. Someone asked me why we mix our health and healing work with something silly like that.

The answer is clear. They are connected. Our body, mind, and spirit are actually all one. For humans to have perfect health, all three components have to be healthy.

In contrast, traditional medicine views health mechanistically, separating the body, mind, and spirit. A medical doctor fixes the body, a psychiatrist fixes the mind, and a pastor fixes the spirit.

We, at The Healing Center, do not view it that way. We take more of a vitalistic view. In our opinion and practice, all healing comes from within our unified, whole self.

- *The Body* needs good nutrition, supplements, herbs, homeopathic medicine, and sometimes prescription medications or surgery.
- *The Mind* needs meditation, calming, emotional releases, and homeopathic remedies.
- *The Spirit* needs God's guidance through prayer, meditation, and counseling.

There are some people who have the gift of inner sight. The Catholic Church calls them seers. The Bible calls them prophets. Some are called mediums because they can "see" and "talk" to those who have died.

Due to my conservative religious upbringing, I always disregarded these things, viewing them as evil or the work of the devil. That is, until I had a patient who had a near-death experience and a face-to-face encounter with God who told her to return to this life and to raise her family. After that, she had vivid psychic visions. Countless times she was able to give her children lifesaving advice.

The people who do readings at The Healing Center are highly spiritual people who have a special connection with their higher power. During a reading, the seer might make some recommendations about the future of the person who is receiving the reading. That person—and all of us in that position—then has the choice to accept and build on that prediction or reject it and choose to do something else. The something else might lead to results better than the prediction.

Case Study: This was the case for BG who came to have a reading at that psychic fair. She had a business that she wanted to sell and asked the reader when it would sell. She was told it would sell in the spring; it was October then.

She decided that was not acceptable. So she started to apply the law of attraction. She created a vision board and worked with it every day. She strongly visualized and imagined that the business had already been sold to a happy, successful new owner who loved doing the work. (Remember, "Already done.") The business deal closed in November.

I believe that the power of her thoughts changed the direction of things. Had BG accepted what the reader said, the sale most likely would have happened in the spring. This shows that we have the ability to greatly influence other parts of our lives as well as our health.

Case Study: One of our patients came to see one of the readers at the same fair. She was told that something was wrong with her husband's rectal area. He had not been having any problems there, but after much nagging by his wife, he finally went to a doctor for a physical. A digital rectal examination and some blood tests showed that he had prostate cancer. He was 41, and this is virtually unheard of at that young age. No doubt, the cancer would have gone undetected for years and perhaps caused his demise. He is now eight years after surgery and doing well.

Sometimes I witness these things and shake my head in disbelief. It is so foreign to my upbringing that it seems unbelievable. But almost daily, I see these wonderful happenings. We might not understand all of this, but it is certainly exciting.

If Life Is a Game, These Are the Rules

If Life Is a Game, These Are the Rules by Cherie Carter-Scott, PhD., contains the following ten rules for being human. I find them to be interesting and thought-provoking.

- You will receive a body. You may like it or hate it, but it will be yours for this entire trip.
- You will learn lessons. You are enrolled in a full-time informal school called "life." Each day in this school, you will have the opportunity to learn lessons. You may like the lessons or think them irrelevant or stupid.
- There are no mistakes, only lessons. Growth is a process of experimentation, of trial and error. The so-called "failed experiments" are as much a part of the process as the experiments that ultimately "work."
- A Lesson is repeated until learned. It will be presented to you in various forms until you have learned it. When you have learned it, you can then go on to the next lesson. If you do not learn easy lessons, they will become harder. You will know you have learned a lesson when your actions change.
- Learning lessons does not end. There is no part of life that does not contain lessons. Every person, every incident is the universal teacher. If you are alive, you have lessons to be learned.
- "There" is no better than "here." Nothing leads to happiness. When your "there" has become "here," you will simply obtain another "there" that again will look better than "here."
- Others are merely mirrors of you. You cannot love or hate something about another person unless it reflects something you love or hate in yourself.
- What you create in your life is up to you. You have all the tools and resources you need; what you do with them is up to you.
- All your answers lie inside you. All you need to do is look, listen, and trust.
- You will forget all of this the moment you are born.

There will be much less stress in the world when we understand these "rules." Natural health is about educating ourselves and learning our lessons. We can either be satisfied with our current state of health or we can learn how to change it. We should not be dependent upon a doctor to fix us. That is our responsibility ... with some coaching from the doctor.

Life and fear of dying

In 2006, Richard Boomer, a local resident of Lakeview, started a news-paper called *Lakeview Area News*. Unfortunately, a few years later, Mr. Boomer died. His family, the editor Linda Huckins, and the staff carried on with the paper for a couple years until they were forced to close.

It is very interesting to observe the lifecycle of an entity such as the *Lakeview Area News*. Like a living thing, the newspaper was born, it came into existence, and it matured and then died. We are born, we mature, and then we pass. There is much debate about the afterlife and also if there is a forelife. There are lively arguments about the concept of reincarnation, past lives, and genetic memory.

There are reports of people who recall near-death experiences, and reports of people who nearly die and do not recall anything. Hundreds of theories exist about what happens to us when we die. Often, a great deal of fear is associated with dying and what will happen to us after we die. Over the years, I have done a lot of work with hospice and I have seen that people's reaction to dying varies a great deal. Some fight to survive and some are ready and peacefully slip away.

It is important to understand that we, like every living entity, have a life-cycle. We were born, and we are going to die. For peace of mind and stress control, we need to spend some time thinking about death. Perhaps we can have peace of mind by reading books about dying and death, counseling with a spiritual advisor, or attending seminars.

My belief is that after we die, part of us carries on. We are much like the newspaper. The physical *Lakeview Area News* died, but an e-mail version kept it going. And then, like with reincarnation, someone else bought the news-paper and it lives again.

Have you noticed that when someone dies, everything and everyone else just continue on? The earth continues to turn. The sun and the stars still shine. People continue to go to their jobs and build new relationships. A part of those who are deceased carries on in the hearts and minds of those who loved them. And from time to time, the name of the person who has passed is spoken. But I believe something more exists. Mostly that belief has been developed by my patients and others who have had near-death experi-ences. The strength of that belief overcomes the fear of dying and generates an excited anticipation. It feels much like being ready to go on a trip or like the night before Christmas.

If you are experiencing fear of dying, it is very important to find peace within. This fear is very stress producing. It will make your body acidic and your life unpleasant. Seek help, use homeopathic remedies or essential oils, read, and seek spiritual counsel. In this way, the rest of your life can be peaceful and joyful.

The Silent Sermon

Someone sent this to me. I found it interesting, thought-provoking, and worth passing on to you. The message of this unknown author is: To be at our best, we need other people, that master mind group.

A member of a certain church, who previously had been attending services regularly, stopped going. After a few weeks, the pastor decided to visit him.

It was a chilly evening. The pastor found the man at home alone, sitting before a blazing fire. Guessing the reason for his pastor's visit, the man welcomed him, led him to a comfortable chair near the fireplace, and waited.

The pastor made himself at home but said nothing. In the grave silence, he contemplated the dance of the flames around the burning logs. After some minutes, the pastor took the fire tongs, carefully picked up a brightly burning ember and placed it to one side of the hearth all alone. Then he sat back in his chair, still silent.

The host watched all this in quiet contemplation. As the one lone ember's flame flickered and diminished, there was a momentary glow and then its fire was no more. Soon it was cold and dead.

Not a word had been spoken since the initial greeting. The pastor glanced at his watch and realized it was time to leave. He slowly stood up, picked up the cold, dead ember and placed it back in the middle of the fire. Immediately it began to glow once more with the light and warmth of the burning coals around it.

As the pastor reached the door to leave, his host spoke up. With a tear running down his cheek, he said, "Thank you so much for your visit and especially for the fiery sermon. I will be back in church next Sunday."

We live in a world, which often tries to say too much with too much talk. Consequently, few listen. Sometimes the best messages are the ones left unspoken.

We humans need the companionship of other people. Facebook and other social networking sites are great, but physical contact is much better. In a group like a church, we find social contact with people of similar religious beliefs as well as a spiritual presence that is greater than the sum of the parts. The joyful feeling that results reduces acidity in our bodies, promoting health and longevity. Stay connected.

Pathology

PATHOLOGY is the science or study of the origin, nature, and course of diseases. It also refers to the condition and processes of a disease and any deviation from a healthy, normal, or efficient condition of the body.

When we think of pathology, it's important to remember the three states of health and illness:

- *Healthy and well* is the condition we all want to be in
- *Functional symptoms* means that we have symptoms but no objective findings appear on medical tests
- *Pathological illness* means that the symptoms have persisted to the point when damage begins to occur, findings show up on medical tests, and diseases with names are diagnosed.

In this chapter, I am going to discuss natural remedies for these pathological conditions.

Cancer prevention begins with your personal choices

The following is information taken from a column by Dr. Mercola.

Cancer rates are increasing in spite of much research by highly technical people and treatment by great specialists. Even the conservative American Cancer Society states that one-third of cancer deaths are linked to poor diet, physical inactivity, and excess weight. Changing our lifestyle can go a very long way toward becoming one less statistic as we aim toward perfect health.

Ways to do this are:

- Normalize your vitamin D3 levels with safe amounts of sun exposure and supplementation if needed. Ask your doctor about testing your vitamin D3 levels.
- Control your insulin levels by limiting your intake of processed

foods and sugars as much as possible. Avoid high fructose corn syrup.

- Get appropriate exercise. Exercise works because it drives insulin levels down.
- Get appropriate amounts of plant-based omega-3 fats.
- Eat according to your blood type and Apo E genetic type. You will read more about the Apo E Gene testing and nutrition later in this book.
- Eat as many vegetables as you comfortably can. Ideally, they should be fresh, organic, raw, or steamed.
- Eat cruciferous vegetables, which are arugula, bok choy, broccoli, Brussels sprouts, cabbage, cauliflower, collards, horseradish, kale, kohlrabi, mustard greens, radish, red cabbage, rutabaga, turnips, turnip greens, and watercress; these have been identified as potent anti-cancer preventers. The brighter the color, the better the vegetable is for you, which is what we mean by "avoid white, eat bright."
- Avoid eating any deep fried foods.
- Maintain an ideal body weight.
- Get enough high-quality sleep.
- Reduce your exposure to environmental toxins like pesticides, household chemical cleaners, synthetic air fresheners, hand sanitizers, and air pollution.
- Never start smoking, stop if you do smoke, and avoid second-hand smoke.
- Use tools to manage stress. Stress can activate a genetic predisposition to develop cancer. The Centers for Disease Control and Prevention (CDC) states that 85 percent of disease is caused by emotions. If this is true, then it is more important than all the other physical things listed here. Make sure that you manage stress. Relaxation, meditation, yoga, tai chi, Emotional Freedom Technique (EFT), and the Silva Method of Mind Development and Stress Control are some tools you can learn. A spiritual practice of your choice is extremely important.

The above are some ways to reduce your cancer risks. There are many more, but these will go a long way toward giving you a good, long healthy life.

Cancer: Physical

So many times when we think about cancer, we focus only on the physical aspects and ignore the mental, emotional, and spiritual. We use chemotherapy and radiation therapy to try to eradicate the abnormal cells that are in the body. It is important to understand that the cancer cells cannot create the environment in which they can live. Cancer is, in that sense, opportunistic. It is an abnormal growth that can only survive in a body with an immune system that does not recognize it as abnormal. Every cell in our body is coded to be recognized as part of the self. But the abnormal cells are allowed to survive when the body's surveillance system is not working correctly. Prevention is our best and easiest treatment, right?

We sometimes inherit a susceptibility to develop cancer. In homeopathy, Dr. Samuel Hahnemann taught us that some people carry a cancer miasm, which is also an inherited susceptibility to develop cancer. Some scientists talk about the cancer gene, but this is not entirely accurate.

So what happens? We might have ancestors who have had cancer. From them, we could have inherited this weakness, this tendency, this susceptibility to develop cancer cells in our own body. A dormant gene might reside in the DNA in our cells. Much like a sleeping lion that is harmless as long as it stays asleep, it can lie silently until something happens to turn it on. What will switch on a dormant gene? What can wake up the sleeping lion and turn it into something unpleasant?

The most common physical reason for activation of these dormant genes is a change in the chemical environment in the cell's nucleus, which is the home of the DNA. We know that cancers thrive in acidic, oxygen-poor places. Cancers are much like rodents. Rats and mice do not like clean, open, lighted places. They like dark, dirty places to nest and hide. What creates the ideal place in which a cancer can survive and thrive? Acidic, toxic areas of the body that have a low level of oxygen.

So, how does this happen?

Our body can become contaminated from:

- toxic exposures from air breathed into the lungs and absorbed through the skin,
- poor quality food,
- internally generated wastes from every cell.

The first thing to do is to stop putting toxic material into your body. The second is to clean up the toxins that are there. And the third is to get proper oxygen to every cell.

Stop eating anything that is not food! Processed items. Sugars, especially high fructose corn syrup. Anything with additives, flowing agents, dyes, and chemicals with names you cannot pronounce.

Pure foods, preferably home grown or home prepared, are the only way to ensure that you are eating real food. Start with making your own yogurt, bread, and soups. Use frozen food, not canned unless you can it yourself. Please do not eat "fast food."

Our body has the ability to eliminate some toxic material, but some toxins are also stored in our fat and muscles. Lack of movement and no exercise reduces our body's ability to remove toxins through our routes of elimination: lungs, skin, kidneys, and liver. Motion in the tissues, vibration from impacts, and contraction of muscles all move internally generated wastes and external toxins from the body. This is why we must move. If we do not move, the fluids around our cells become like a swamp rather than a cool fresh stream.

Avoiding trans fats will ensure that our cell membranes are more able to transport oxygen into the cells. Grass-fed beef and wild game contain about two percent trans fats. Feedlot beef can have as high as 40 percent trans fats. The same is true of wild-caught versus farm-raised fish. When we fool with nature, we often mess it up.

Detoxing or cleansing toxins from the body is of extreme importance to help remove stored wastes. You could get some professional advice about cleansing. If you are not healthy, you must build the body first before doing a lot of detoxing. There are many safe ways to do this, but exercise is actually the most important and the most natural.

Eat only real food and get your body moving.

Cancer: Mental

Most of us do not even think about the mental aspects of cancer treatment.

First, there is the shock of bad news about a diagnosis of cancer. Many people tell me they feel like they were punched in the stomach or they felt their heart stop. For some, they are already dead in their minds.

We use a homeopathic remedy, Gelsemium 200C, taken twice daily for five days to remove the shock of this bad news. This can be taken at any time after the diagnosis is given, but the sooner the better, to help a person think more clearly as they find their way through this life-changing experience. Family members can take this remedy as well.

People diagnosed with cancer often experience an immediate fear of death, and some immediately begin to prepare for death. This is a conditioned response. This is unfortunately much like a superstition. Some people think of Friday, the 13th, as an unlucky day or that crossing the path of a black cat is an unlucky event. We logically know that these things are not necessarily unlucky, but we have just been programmed to think that way. The same is true for certain diagnoses like cancer.

Dr. Carlos M. Garcia, MD, has written a book titled *Cancer Is a Symptom*, which explains how we have to learn to think differently about this disease. If we can modify our thinking, then we can come to see ridding our body of cancer as no more difficult to correct than resolving a case of bad bronchitis. One of the challenges is overcoming the old programming about the severity of this condition.

I'm sure almost all of us know people who have been diagnosed with cancer but have survived and lived for a long time. I personally know many miraculous stories of recovery. We think of these as "miraculous" because we often do not know the cause behind the recovery.

Learn to be happy all the time, change the things in your life that you need to change and let go of the things you cannot fix. Let go of those things that you have no control of such as the government, the health care system, Medicare, the President, your past, your relatives, etc. Let it go. Fix your world, let go of the rest. Stop watching the news. The negatives just create more acidity. Focus on your future perfect health. You cannot serve two masters, the past and the future. You must choose where to put your energy, either into the sunshine of the future or the darkness of the past.

A very important part of recovery from any illness, cancer included, is our mental state. So, even if you've been diagnosed with cancer, think about how old you want to be when you pass over and then see yourself driving and dancing until that day. Think of your upcoming years like miles ahead of you down the road. If you use your GPS, you must type in an address. You have to know where you want to go. That is like your life. Without a program of perfect health until some age of your choice, you cannot get there. Learn to think perfect health, even with the stress of a painful diagnosis. Remember: You become what you think about most of the time.

Cancer: Emotional

Many years ago my mentor, Dr. Bennett, said "cancers might be caused by what we eat, but more often they are caused by what eats at us." Many times, we carry emotions, often from our childhood that we are not aware of, or we keep them hidden out of sight.

Louise Hay wrote a book called *You Can Heal Your Life*. After 15 years of working as a counselor, she noticed that physical illness is often associated with emotional conditions. For example, she noticed that liver and gallbladder disease are often associated with anger, bitterness, and resentment. She found that people who have chronic back problems often have lack of support and/or lack of financial support. Bladder problems were connected to people who were "pissed off" all the time. Throat conditions were aggravated by not speaking one's mind. And so on.

> **Case Study:** Often, these hidden emotions are the result of conflicts that we have with other people. Six or seven years ago, I had a patient with stage IV breast cancer who was carrying a deep resentment toward her husband who had been unfaithful to her ten years before. After she was able to totally forgive him and let go of her resentment and anger, the cancer disappeared with no additional treatment and she is cancer free today.

O. Carl Simonton, radiation oncologist and teacher of visualization healing, said that people who live or work in an environment that they hate are more likely to have serious illnesses. His advice: Either find new work or living conditions or change your mind about the situation. You have to be happy.

Our bodies know how to be perfectly healthy, but something might interfere with that, causing disease. I often prescribe a tool called Emotional Releasing. The protocol is to create a timeline of every emotionally traumatic event that you can recall. Yes, you've heard me emphasize this before—as well as the release letter below. And I'm going to do so again because it is so important.

Here is a list of events that can cause trapped emotions: grief, loss of love, abandonment, humiliation, fright, bad news, worry, disappointment, anger, homesickness, jealousy, dishonesty, and I'm sure there are more. Using one event at a time, write a letter to the person involved. This letter is for your own healing and will never be sent to that person. It is not their problem; it is yours. In the letter, write everything you wish you could say to that person. When you finish writing, add an ending that states, "I will no longer carry your debt for you physically, mentally, emotionally, or spiritually." And then add, "I love you. I bless you. I release you. And I forgive you for everything I think you have done to me." Read this letter out loud three times and then burn it. As you watch the smoke and flame, release this negative emotion to your higher power. Then, in a week or so, think about that situation again. If it is not completely resolved, write another letter. Do this until it is gone.

Keep doing this with every traumatic event on the timeline until you have cleaned up as much of the old garbage as you can remember. You will experience an amazing peacefulness and lightness of being.

Tapping techniques, like those described in *The Happiness Code* by Gary Laundre, are very valuable to release trapped emotions. These techniques use acupuncture points and the meridian energy system to tap into and heal the stuck emotional condition. Homeopathic and Bach Flower remedies have been used for a long time to help eliminate trapped negative emotions. Emotional release massages are another amazing tool to release old emotions so they no longer poison the physical body. Meditating on what you desire for your future will create that outcome, unless you sabotage it.

Clean up your old, outdated emotions.

Cancer: Spiritual

So many times when we treat cancer, we focus only on the physical aspects and ignore the other aspects. We use chemotherapy and radiation therapy to try to eradicate the abnormal cells that are in the body. But we forget about the spiritual.

When we are children, we feel like we will live forever. We do not think much about death and dying. The reality is that we are mortal beings with a physical body that will wear out someday and cease to function. With any potentially life-threatening condition, we are forced to face our mortality—the death of our body

Yet another component of life is that we are, first and foremost, spiritual beings who are experiencing the physical world of apparent objective reality through our physical senses. If you are totally focused on your physical world, this might be hard to understand. Indeed, it has taken me many years to get some sort of understanding about how all this works. With that being said, there are times when I know that things are much different than I think they are.

For what it's worth, I will share my philosophy on this. You can take from it what you will. Like a friend of mine says, "When you eat fruit, just eat the meaty part and spit out the seeds and pulp."

A spiritual being resides within us and is that part of us that is our awareness of being. If we stop everything for a few minutes, close our eyes, and repeat the words, "I am," a few times, we become aware of being. This awareness of being is our spiritual self, the part of us that controls the direction of our physical lives. This is the voice of God. This is the intuition that often guides us with inner vision, the still small voice, and the gut feelings.

In contrast to that we have our ego! The ego is the part of our mind that wants to run everything and get the credit for doing it. It is the part that competes for glory and wants the thrill of excitement and adventure. Ego often guides us to make the "wrong decision for the wrong reasons."

Cancer is a physical condition in which certain cells in our body have lost their self-control. Each cell is supposed to have a self-regulating mechanism, controlled by its DNA, that programs it to die at a certain time. Each tissue type has a specific life cycle, much like any organism. Old cells die; new cells come in to take their place. That's the way of life in a healthy body.

Programmed cell death is called *apoptosis*. Each cell in a tissue type lives a predetermined length of time and then it dies. For example, blood cells live only a few days whereas nerve cells live for years.

Sometimes, a protein appears on the cell membrane called ENOX2 proteins. These prevent the natural programmed cell death from occurring. As new cells begin to accumulate, they grow into masses and tumors.

It is my belief that our spiritual part, our awareness of being, is here for a purpose. When we follow that purpose, spiritual evolution occurs. When our spiritual being no longer has a purpose or when its purpose is completed, the spirit begins to find ways for the physical body to release it. It knows that the physical body must die so the spirit can be released.

Cancer is one way for that to happen. I have seen this many times. When people have no purpose, they begin to deteriorate. But they can regenerate if they regain a purpose for living. I have seen people come back from the brink to total recovery and go on to live long, purpose-filled lives.

The outcome, one way or the other, all comes down to what messages we are sending to our spiritual self. Are we purposefully caring for our physical body, avoiding toxins and feeding it properly? What are we mentally envisioning, saying to ourselves, and feeling about ourselves? What are our emotions? What message is that spiritual part of us getting? Life is great or life sucks?

When our spiritual part, the awareness of being, can no longer learn from the physical experiences of the body, it is time to go. Then our spiritual part will create an exit point. It is my belief that these occur every ten years or so. Many people experience near fatal injuries, accidents, and illness every ten to 15 years. It is interesting to note that people who live purposefully rarely experience that.

We must let go of our old thinking. We must remove our old misconceptions about life. To return to perfect health after a diagnosis of cancer, we must have a purpose that is worthwhile for ourselves, our family, our immediate community, and perhaps the rest of humanity. Every night before going to sleep, we must envision our life the way we want it to be, even if we are facing a serious life-threatening illness. This is faith. Unless our awareness of being understands clearly the purpose for continuing our physical existence, our life cannot and will not go on.

Do not pray for healing. Praying for healing is weak; it is like trying; it is not doing. Do not pray for cancer to be removed. Pray for perfect physical health so you can fulfill your purpose for living.

Then state your purpose. Be definite. Why do you want to live? Why is it imperative that you live? What is so important that you must remain here in physical form? You have to be very convincing. You cannot be like a whining child. You must be sure, assertive, and even a little pushy. Think like this just before you go to sleep until you achieve a feeling as if it is already done.

Do not tell anyone else what you are doing, thinking, and praying. Your request must be done in secret—between you, your awareness of being, and God. When you tell others, they will fill you with doubt and fear. There is no room for doubt and fear. You are not negotiating, deal making, or begging. You are making a clear statement of definite purpose. Praying in this manner is creative. By praying in this way, your desired outcome is granted.

Jesus said, "If you have faith like a grain of mustard seed, nothing will be impossible for you." When we think spiritually in this manner, something changes in our DNA and the ENOX2 proteins are removed from the cells. Then the normal programmed cell death of the cancerous cells begins to occur and your own body removes the tumors so you can return to perfect health with a new purpose for living.

Leaky gut syndrome

Leaky gut syndrome is a condition that traditional medicine does not recognize as legitimate. The underlying premise is that the "pores" in the lining of the small bowel become damaged and begin to allow large particles of partially digested food to enter the blood. When this happens, your body begins to make antibodies against these "foreign" particles. This is the basis for food allergies and some of the auto-immune diseases that we experience.

For example, casein is a large protein molecule in milk. To get nutritional value from this protein, the body has to break it down into amino acids. When you drink milk, the hydrochloric acid in your stomach converts pepsinogen, which is a pre-enzyme, to the enzyme pepsin, which breaks down the casein into polypeptides. The polypeptides are moved into the small intestine, called the duodenum. There, protease enzymes from the pancreas break down the polypeptides into peptides and finally into amino acids.

If the polypeptides or the peptides get absorbed into the blood before they are fully digested into amino acids, antibodies begin to form because these are not supposed to be there in the blood stream. Nasal congestion, post nasal drainage, headaches, fibromyalgia, joint pain, irritable bowel syndrome, gastro esophageal reflux, irritable bladder, and many more symptoms can develop.

The most common cause of leaky gut syndrome is an over growth of yeast, such as Candida albicans, in the intestines. This yeast is normally present in the end of the small intestine, the terminal ileum. Its purpose there is to clean up any undigested sugars that make it through the small bowel. Too much sugar entering the colon, however, will cause fermentation, gas, bloating, irritable bowel, and other unpleasantries.

Reduce sugars and starches. The yeast can only use sugar as its food source. Taking probiotics, which are beneficial bacteria, will seed new, healthy, normal flora back into that ecosystem. Avoiding antibiotics will reduce the likelihood of loss of bowel flora. Also avoid chlorine, fluoride, steroids, cortisone, and hormones because they cause die-off of the good bugs. Use a bowel or colon cleanse at least once a year; twice per year for some people. Then the lining of the bowel can return to normal, removing all the symptoms of the leaky gut syndrome.

I'll present more on Candida and good intestinal bugs later in the Natural Treatments part of this book

Chronic fatigue

It is normal to be full of energy and vitality. Why are so many people tired all the time?

Chronic fatigue has many causes. Some are allergies, often to food; unresolved viral infections; unresolved grief; illnesses like diabetes, hypothyroidism, liver disease, kidney failure, heart disease; toxins from environment and yeast by-products; and hormone imbalances.

Case Study: RN had chronic nasal allergies, was tired all the time, and had irritable bowel syndrome. There were two steps to his recovery. First, I instructed him to determine any food allergies by using the "eliminate, challenge, and observe" process along with the Eat Right for Your Blood Type program. This gave him much improvement, but he still had a lot of lingering fatigue and post nasal drainage. So he had a colon cleanse that almost totally cleared up both the post nasal drainage and the energy drain. This indicated that the food allergies were aggravated by a poorly functioning bowel.

Dr. D'Adamo, in *Eat Right for Your Type,* and Caroline Sutherland, in *Your Body Knows,* teach us that inflammatory foods are a huge factor in chronic fatigue. The five most common food groups that cause inflammation are dairy, wheat, corn, eggs, and foods that contain yeast or fungi.

I know I've described the "eliminate, challenge, and observe" process earlier, but I'll repeat it now because it's relevant here. First, eliminate one food group for two weeks, then check how you feel. Next, challenge your system by eating from that food group for one day. Then observe what happens within your body over the next four days. If your body reacts to eliminating one or more food groups from your diet, you might begin to see subtle or dramatic changes in your health.

You also can do a pulse test to help with food selection.

Chronic fatigue has many causes. When seeking a remedy, good nutrition is a first place to start. Sometimes, cleansing and detox programs are needed to clean things up a bit. And sometimes, special remedies are needed to build your body's natural healing mechanisms.

Gastro esophageal reflux disease (GERD)

A patient recently asked some questions about acid reflux, known as gastro esophageal reflux disease (GERD).

To explain the mechanics of GERD, let me begin with how we are put together. The esophagus is a muscular tube that delivers food from the mouth through the chest cavity to the stomach. It enters the abdominal cavity through an opening in the diaphragm called the diaphragmatic hiatus, which is the site of a condition known as a hiatal hernia. This opening acts like a valve to prevent backwash of food and liquid up into the esophagus.

When we eat, the parietal cells in the stomach release a surge of hydrochloric acid. This acid is needed to convert the pre-enzyme pepsinogen into pepsin, which then is used to reduce protein into polypeptides, which later are broken down into peptides then to amino acids the body can use.

The lining of the stomach is covered with a layer of mucus to protect it from the stomach acid. During the acid surge, the acid in the stomach is about as caustic as battery acid. While the lining on the stomach walls can handle this level of acidity, the lining of the esophagus does not have the necessary protective mucus. Acidic juice from the stomach refluxing back up into the unprotected esophagus is what causes most of the problems with GERD, including that feeling of having an inflated balloon in the upper part of your chest and throat.

Causes of GERD might be hereditary due to a genetically weak valve or weak esophageal muscles. But mostly, however, the malady usually originates from particular body functions. This is why I say that gastro esophageal reflux disease is another one of those man-made diseases that is related to our modern culture, food, and eating practices.

Coughing and lifting while bending will intermittently push the stomach up through the hiatus, stretching and weakening the valve action of the hiatus. A big belly will mechanically push the stomach up through the hiatus when lying down or bending over. If your meal is too large, there will not be enough enzymes to pre-digest all the protein and some of it will begin to putrefy, causing gas. This will create back pressure on the hiatus, pushing liquids up into the esophagus. Gas-forming yeast and bacteria might also be a contributing factor. Nicotine, caffeine, alcohol, and stress all cause acid production when no food is present, contributing to this problem. We have seen many cases of GERD completely resolve with elimination of milk and all processed dairy products.

Some people with GERD, especially the older crowd, actually do not have enough acid in their stomachs. You can determine if your stomach is producing too much or too little acid by doing the following: Take a teaspoon of apple cider vinegar at the beginning of a meal. If that helps eliminate the sensation of heartburn, then you need to add acid to your digestive system. Use Betine HCl prior to the meal to increase acid. Betine HCl is a supplement found in most health stores. It is the same as the hydrochloric acid produced by your stomach. If the vinegar makes you feel worse, then you know that you have too much acid.

Some people attempt to control GERD symptoms with pharmaceutically manufactured proton pump inhibitors (PPIs) like Prilosec, Prevacid, and Nexium. These medications can block up to 90 percent of the stomach acid production. That is good if you have a bleeding ulcer that needs to be healed, but if stomach acid is blocked too much and for too long, our body cannot digest proteins into amino acids. Because amino acids are the building blocks of all body structures, not having enough of them is like building a house with only 50 percent of the required lumber. Not good. Rebound hyperacidity, osteoporosis, and reaction with other meds are just a few of the conditions being warned about due to long-term use of PPIs.

Blocking stomach acid with the much-advertised "purple pill" and other PPIs is not very healthy, long term. In fact, the pharmaceutical manufacturers recommend taking those products for a maximum of 28 days. If you must temporarily block stomach acid, it would be safer to use an H2 blocker like Zantac or Pepcid. But these have long-term problems also. If you do need these, take them at bedtime for a few weeks. This way, night time acid production is blocked to protect the stomach and esophagus when you are lying down, but it will not block acid at meal times.

As is so often true with optimal healing, it is best to fix the underlying problem instead of covering it up by treating just the symptom. The Blood Type diet and/or elimination of all milk and processed dairy and wheat products have been helpful for many of our patients.

Try this for two weeks. Then challenge your body to see what happens.

- Reduce the quantity of food in your meals.
- Avoid grazing all day long.
- To heal esophagitis, take one teaspoon of aloe vera juice, undiluted, four times a day; this has been miraculous in many cases.
- Occasionally use Tums or a little baking soda to help with heartburn, but too much or too often will cause rebound hyper acidity. This means when the acid comes back it might be worse than before. Avoid Maalox, Mylanta, Gaviscon, and other aluminum containing antacids. Aluminum is allegedly a factor in the development of Alzheimer's disease.
- Take probiotics, such as acidophilus, to help reduce gas-forming yeast.
- Take digestive enzymes with pepsin, amylase, lipase, and protease to assist with digesting foods.

- Eat fiber and activated charcoal to absorb toxins in the food that might be causing problems.
- Use herbal Slippery Elm to cool a hot digestive tract.
- Prop the head of your bed up four inches and use gravity to prevent back-wash into your esophagus at night.
- Reduce the size of your waist to reduce physical pressure on the diaphragm.
- Use a liver cleanse every four to six months; this is highly beneficial.
- If you have a hiatal hernia, use the heel drop technique[1] or abdominal massage[2] to bring the stomach back into the abdominal cavity.

There are many answers to GERD besides blocking all the natural acids that your body needs for proper digestion. Look beyond the purple pill.

Irritable bowel syndrome (IBS)

Irritable bowel syndrome (IBS) is a term that was coined a number of years ago in regard to people who complained of abdominal pain, constipation, and diarrhea, however when they went to a doctor to have tests and x-rays, everything appeared to be normal. IBS is also call spastic colon, colitis, or functional bowel syndrome.

Practitioners of traditional medicine expect to see a cause that shows up as an abnormality in lab tests, x-rays, or something physically wrong in the body in order to make a diagnosis and prescribe treatment. Unfortunately, many times these problems are functional. That means they express symptoms and aches and pains but no physical abnormality that a doctor can find. Sometimes, people are told to see the psychiatrist because there is nothing wrong physically. Unfortunately, I have done that myself in former times.

---

1 A hiatal hernia occurs when part of the stomach slides up into the chest cavity. This causes chest pain, shortness of breath, and heartburn. The heel drop technique is to: Drink eight ounces of water, then stand on your tip toes, then drop onto your heels with knees straight. This action will pull the stomach back down into the abdominal cavity. I have actually heard a sucking, popping sound when it comes back down. You might have to do this several times.

2 Abdominal massage can also be used when part of the stomach is up in the chest cavity. Abdominal massage is this: Sit in a chair, leaning backward at about a 45 degree angle. Then push up with your thumbs into the central upper abdomen, which is the V-shaped area between your ribs. Dig your thumbs into this soft area and gently pull downward while forcefully exhaling all your breath. Sometimes you can feel the stomach pulled tightly up against the diaphragm. Do this repeatedly until you feel relief as the stomach goes back down into the abdominal cavity.

In natural and homeopathic medicine, however, the symptom itself is a warning that something is wrong. We should not put a band-aid on it to make it go away. We should not suppress it with pharmaceutical drugs. We should cleanse and build the body's natural healing mechanism through homeopathic remedies, herbs, and essential oils so the whole person can get better.

Many times, IBS can be fixed by controlling food intake. We have seen good results by eliminating dairy products and wheat from the diet. Following the Eat Right for Your Blood Type program almost always fixes IBS. Very gentle cleanses and the herbal remedies Slippery Elm, Marshmallow, Dandelion, Licorice Root, and many others have been successfully used to relieve IBS.

If you have this problem, do not give up. Rather, try some natural and nutritional remedies to get back to perfect health.

Irritable bladder syndrome or interstitial cystitis (IC)

Irritable bladder syndrome, which is also known as interstitial cystitis (IC), is another functional condition that traditional medicine finds difficult to deal with.

Cystitis means bladder inflammation. Usually, this is associated with infection and is easily treated with herbs and prescription medications. Interstitial refers to the tissue of the bladder lining. So the term interstitial cystitis literally means inflammation of the lining of the bladder when no infection is involved.

The symptoms are, however, usually the same as one would experience with urinary tract infection (UTI). Burning with urination, bladder pain and spasms, urgency to void, frequency, and sometimes leaking are the aggravating symptoms of IC.

Traditional treatment involves instilling medications into the bladder through a catheter and oral medications, which are immune suppressors. Often, these work to relieve the symptoms but do nothing to actually fix the underlying cause. They are costly, time consuming, and inconvenient.

The first line of natural treatment has to do with dietary intake. Remember this condition is caused by inflammation of the bladder lining. So, inflammatory food and chemicals must be strictly avoided. Caffeine in all forms, that is, coffee, tea, and chocolate, are very inflammatory. Nicotine, again in all forms, affects the bladder. Food additives, sugar, and alcohol can be culprits. All artificial sweeteners, such as Splenda and NutraSweet, are known to cause inflammation in the bladder. Lectins, which are remnants of the immune systems of plants and animals, are in our food and can be inflammatory.

Stress is a factor because it causes a break down in our weakest system. This weak link might be caused by genetic factors, recurrent infections, trauma such as holding urine too long, or new and old emotional events. Treating stress with prescription medication can be somewhat helpful but, many times, these have side effects. Learning relaxation and meditation is the preferred way to manage stress.

Herbal medications like Nature's Sunshine Products JPX and Urinary Maintenance have been helpful to nourish the bladder tissues. We have also seen excellent results with Dr. Peter D'Adamo's Blood Type diet. The "avoid" foods on the blood type lists should be eliminated completely for two to three months on a trial basis.

Capsules or teas made from the following herbs might be very helpful:

- Corn silk, which has soothing and diuretic properties.
- Horsetail, which is an astringent and mild diuretic with tissue-healing properties.
- Marshmallow Root, which has soothing anti-inflammatory properties. Marshmallow is best as a cold tea; soak the herb in cold water for several hours, strain, and drink.

Homeopathic remedies Causticum, Cantharis, and Staphysagria have all been highly beneficial for dealing with the underlying causes of the inflammation in the lining of the bladder. It is important to try some of these natural things before or while taking the traditional treatments.

Both irritable bladder syndrome and interstitial cystitis have some roots in blocked meridian and chakra energy. Squatting exercise, yoga, meditation, energy clearing, and emotional releasing are often very helpful.

Joint pain

Not all joint pain is related to arthritis, but that is what we tend to call it. The most common joint pains are caused by wear and tear of the cartilages, ligaments, and tendons that hold the joints together. All of these tissues are made of collagen. The collagen tissues have poor blood supply and tend to repair themselves very slowly. The most important part of repairing and healing the collagen tissue is to have in our diet all the ingredients needed to make collagen.

To make collagen, our body goes through a series of chemical steps. The results of two of these steps are chondroitin and glucosamine. If we add these directly to our diet, we can increase the production of collagen and repair our cartilages faster. Dietary sources of chondroitin and glucosamine are gelatin and animal cartilage or gristle from meat. Most of us do not eat enough gelatin and most throw away the disgusting cartilage. So adding a supplement containing these will be very helpful. However, and this is important, avoid chondroitin if you have a high PSA or prostate cancer.

The third ingredient needed is methylsulfonylmethane (MSM). This is an excellent source of dietary sulfur that helps break down the damaged collagen so it can be repaired.

The fourth ingredient is omega-3 from fish oil or flax seed oil or chia seeds. Omega-3 acts as an anti-inflammatory and also helps in the production of lubricating gel in the joints. Another great source of raw material to make the lubricating gel is hyaluronic acid. We like the brand name product Baxyl, which has a unique protective process so it is not broken down by the digestive juices in the stomach and small intestine.

High antioxidant fruit supplements like Noni Juice, Thai Go, and Xango are very helpful in the temporary reduction of inflammation in the joints. I say temporary because the body needs to have the building blocks of chondroitin, glucosamine, MSM, and omega-3 to repair the cartilage and get permanent relief from joint pain. These should also be balanced with a good nutritional program like Eat Right for Your Blood Type.

Homeopathic medications are also very helpful with joint pain. Arnica is fabulous for sprains, strains, and acute injuries of the joints. There are many other remedies for chronic joint pains. To determine the remedy best for you, consult with someone skilled in homeopathy regarding your symptoms as well as other health issues.

Bone spurs or calcium deposits

Lots of people have bone spurs in their necks, back, shoulders, knees, heels, and other joints. Development of these spurs is a long-term process, and it can take up to 20 years of chronic inflammation in a soft tissue, like a tendon, to form a spur made from calcium. The traditional medical thinking is that spurs can only be removed with surgery. This is simply not true and I have many happy patients to prove it.

Case Study: Several years ago, I saw a gentleman in the office who had spurs in his neck. About three months before, these were visible on x-ray and were causing him a lot of discomfort in his neck and down his arms. I recommended that he take herbal Hydrangea root, which is known to dissolve soft tissue calcium, calcified stones, and bone spurs, along with a homeopathic remedy Calcerea Carbonicum 6C. His neck pain was gone after seven to ten days, and after three months of this treatment, the spurs were no longer visible on the x-ray.

This is amazing to me! It shows just how much bone is dynamic, how it is constantly being broken down and built back up. I am not sure this will work for every case of spurs, but it is worth a try. The cost of Hydrangea root and homeopathic Calcerea Carbonicum 6C is around $30.00 per month for three to six months. If you take the herbal Hydrangea for more than month, take a vacation from it by using it only six days a week or days 1 through 25 of each month.

Joint pain and food sensitivities

This is the unedited story, written by one woman about her journey with food allergies, arthritis, and her desire for help with bone spurs.

Fifteen years ago, I had pain from neck to toe. Was diagnosed with osteoarthritis and told that I could feel encouraged because of the great advancements in joint replacements. I told the rheumatologist that I was hopeful it wouldn't get to that, and she predicted that I would be in a wheelchair in ten years if I wasn't willing to consider joint replacements.

I went on a 7-day Sonne's fast and cleanse [a fasting program from Sonne's Organic Foods] and all pain disappeared. I added foods back very carefully and over time (and a couple more fasts) discovered what gave me pain: wheat, dairy, carrots, lemons, soy, and safflower oil. Since then I have controlled my diet and have taken Glucos-amine sulfate, and Chondroitin sulfate. No joint replacements yet.

I took up bike riding last year. I work as a school counselor in a large two-story building and am up and down stairs all day with no difficulty. So, I think my food avoidance has worked well for me.

I did suffer a recurrence of symptoms some years back and after weeks of puzzlement, and distortions to my finger joints, I discovered that stearic acid in tablets and capsules is a problem for me. [Author's Note: Stearic acid is a flowing agent used by the manufacturer to effi-ciently move powders through the tablet and capsule making equip-ment. Some labels will show talc and magnesium stearate, which are also flowing agents.]

When the attack of thumb arthritis hit a few months ago, I had not changed anything, or so I thought, for three weeks of pain. Finally, in desperation, it occurred to me that one of my supplements could have changed. When I went through them, reading every label, I discovered that the Carlson people had added safflower oil to the vitamin D I had taken for years. I immediately stopped taking it and the pain subsided within a day. Soon after, I ate one of Pame-la's Ginger Cookies (Pamela's products had been a trusted friend for years) and I experienced thumb pain. Read the label to find safflower oil. Same experience with Trader Joe's Black Bean Enchiladas, Food for Life's China Black Rice Bread, and virtually all the baked goods from the gluten-free bakery I have frequented for six years. The way I see it, I could tolerate small amounts of that wretched oil, but when I ingested a dose every day, my immune system reacted.

However, right after discovering the oil in my vitamin D3, I purchased a roasted chicken from my local market so that I could have easy meals during a busy week at school. Thumb pain all week. Stopped eating the chicken and pain subsided. I asked them if they used safflower oil on their roasted chickens and they said no. I didn't believe them. Last week, feeling a cold coming on, I put together a pot of chicken soup, using Pacific's Organic Chicken Broth and organic chicken thighs. Pain after one bowl. So, chicken is on my list of avoid foods.

The bone spurs are not pleasant, but are not horrible when I stay away from offending foods. Yesterday my pain seemed to be from more than just the spurs. Was it the beef I ate for lunch? Was it the bike ride and over use of that spur laden joint? My body seems to sing when I eat salmon, so I'll try to keep to that all week. Love it but anything gets tiresome over time. Do you have any suggestions?

I recommended that she take herbal Hydrangea one capsule three times per day for days 1 through 25 of each month for three to four months with homeopathic Calcerea Carbonicum 6C, one pellet dissolved in the mouth once per day, for the spurs in her hands and thumbs.

Here is her unedited feedback:

Hi, Bob,

I wrote you back in May about the pain/bone spur at the base of my thumb. I did the hydrangea root through June, August, and am back on it for October. Have continued the Calcerea Carbonicum, but sometimes forget to take it. Thumb pain much better and, surprisingly, Heberdeen's Nodules [these are the little bumps on the joints below your fingernails] are much smaller.

It took them over ten years to develop to the mounds they were, so I should expect the process of reducing their size will be slow. My hands are much more flexible, and it seems the skin on the second knuckles of my fingers seems more wrinkled, suggesting that the knuckle has become smaller, leaving slightly baggy skin. Still, have fleeting pain in my left thumb joint, and it continues to seem bigger than before. But I am much better and can ride my road bike for many miles without trouble.

Thank you, thank you.

I share these letters to illustrate how the foods we eat can cause inflammation in our genetically weakest system.

This is a great example of how something as simple as your food can make you ill or well. It also clearly points out the effectiveness of some simple supplements. So pay attention. You might also be affected by the foods you eat.

There are a few dietary things to consider if you have problems with bone spurs. Calcium carbonate is a big culprit in this problem. That is what causes "hardness" in water. It is the scale that builds up in a tea kettle, coffee pot, shower/tub, and on other hard surfaces. It is the type of calcium in Tums and many calcium supplements. Too much of this will cause hardening in our body. It is better to use calcium citrate for your calcium supplementation.

Too much acidity in our systems also is a problem. The acidity increases the formation of calcium deposits in inflamed areas of our body. Areas of the body that are inflamed from injury or from eating foods that contain lectin are targets for calcium deposits. This is true especially when the body's acid levels are high. Some medications increase acidity. For example, Ibuprofen (Motrin) is an anti-inflammatory, but it also increases acidity, so it can indirectly add to the inflammation issues.

So avoid acidic foods, sugar, tomatoes, oranges, pork, pop, and so on. Follow your food sensitivity list, the Eat Right for Your Blood Type program, or the Apo E Gene diet. But most of all, learn to listen to your own body. The Blood Type diet is a guideline only. Learn to muscle test yourself to see what is good for you. Drink lots of good, pure water. And use medications only if needed.

Chronic low back pain

Chronic low back pain is one of the most common complaints we see in a busy medical office. It is the most common reason that people lose time at work.

Most back problems begin with an injury of some sort, something that sets the stage for an ongoing problem later. It could be a childhood event, an accident, loss of muscular strength and conditioning, or a deficiency in the material needed to make cartilage and bone.

The natural approach to chronic low back pain has multiple steps. If there is an acute injury, begin with homeopathic Arnica and see your friendly chiropractor or massage therapist as soon as possible.

If the initial injury is old, it is still important to take homeopathic Arnica 30C daily for about one week. This will remove the shock from the original injury that is still stored in your connective tissue and muscle.

Next, add supplements that nourish bone and connective tissue. Bioplasma is a cell salt combination that contains 12 basic ingredients needed to rebuild these tissues. The combination of chondroitin, glucosamine, and MSM has been found to be highly effective in creating new cartilage and other connective tissue. However, men should not take chondroitin if they have prostate issues. Minerals like calcium, magnesium, phosphorus, boron, and other trace minerals are very important. Add Mineral Chi or Ionic Minerals from NSP or some other balanced colloidal or ionic mineral supplement.

If the injury is older than five years, it has probably caused formation of bone spurs in the inflamed ligaments and tendons. Herbal Hydrangea, one capsule three times per day for one month, with homeopathic Calcerea Carbonicum 6C, one pellet per day for three months, has been shown to break down bone spurs in the older injuries. If that does not work, you can substitute homeopathic Hekla Lava 6C for the Calcerea Carbonicum and repeat the Hydrangea for one month. Use the Hydrangea on days 1 through 25 if you use it for multiple months. Chronic daily use might decrease the effectiveness of some herbal medications.

Also start a careful general conditioning program. At first, do this under some sort of supervision such as physical therapy, a personal trainer, or a fitness center. Chiropractic adjustments should be a part of this program as you attempt to re-educate the structural elements of your body to remember what they are supposed to do.

Strengthening the weak muscle of the abdomen and back are essential for a healthy back. Walking and swinging the arms is a fundamental part for rebuilding the back. Do this at least one month for every year you have had chronic back pain.

Osteoporosis or brittle bones

Osteoporosis is a serious health issue that causes lots of suffering and might compromise one's overall health, leading to death earlier than expected.

The current treatment recommends use of the prescription medications in the bisphosphonate family: Fosamax, Actonel, and Boniva. The unfortunate part of this treatment is that it is likely to cause a serious bone condition called osteonecrosis, which means dead bone. These medications work by replacing part of the bone with an inert material that delays the breakdown of bone thereby slowing osteoporosis, but they do not build new bone. The problem is that, over time, this inert or dead material will make the bones more brittle. The worse news is that it stays in the bone for 18 months up to ten years. Current medical guidelines suggest use of these medications for no more than five years because this treatment can cause brittle bone. Hmm. Then what are you supposed to do?

You might want to read a fascinating story that broke on National Public Radio in 2009. It was titled "How a Bone Disease Grew to Fit the Prescription" and written by Alix Spiegel. Google this if you are interested. It seems that a particular pharmaceutical company hired an advertising agency to create a name for a new disease, which they named Osteopenia. This was literally done to create a bigger market for one of their already-existing products. This story will give you some insight into how a medicine can be recommended by your doctor, yet he might not really know the whole story.

Natural treatment for osteoporosis must include exercise. I once saw a 14-year-old boy with osteoporosis in his leg after a fracture that was treated with no weight bearing for six weeks. Bone needs stimulation from low impact of mild to moderate exercise.

Elimination of acid-producing foods, such as pork, pop, sugar, fruit juice with sugar added, processed dairy products, potatoes, and tomatoes, is a must if you are facing osteoporosis. An interesting statistic is that the three countries with the highest consumption of processed milk are United States, Australia, and Sweden, and they also have the highest osteoporosis rates. Hmm. That is probably not just a coincidence. Homogenizing milk releases an enzyme, xanthine oxidase, that is very acidic and is not present in raw dairy.

Calcium citrate, 500 mg, with magnesium, 250 mg, three times per day gives adequate absorbable calcium. Vitamin D3, 4000 to 6000 IUs per day, is needed for healthy bone.

There are many skeletal support products on the market for additional minerals. Bioplasma, a product by Hyland's, is a combination of 12 cell salts, all of which support structural tissues. Homeopathic Symphytum 30C, one per week, will help heal any micro-fractures that are occurring. Homeopathic Calcerea Carbonicum 6C or homeopathic Hekla Lava 6C, one pellet once per day, with herbal Hydrangea will reduce bone spurs and enhance the deposition of calcium back into normal bone.

All of these things support the natural production of bone and none interfere with normal physiology of bone like the prescription medication.

I will give further details about Bioplasma in a later section about feeding the body with proper nutrition.

Sinus trouble

Many people complain of sinus problems. I used to be one of them. I never had any nasal congestion or itchy eyes until I came to Michigan. Then, slowly over the years, things got so bad that, in the early 1990s, I was taking antibiotics at least eight times a year for sinus infections. I had become sensitive to everything.

Three days after I went to work for Dr. Grant Born, DO, at the Born Clinic in Grand Rapids, he said to me, "You have food allergies and Candida! I am tired of hearing you sniffing all the time. You need to fix that." I was amazed. He knew without an examination what was wrong. I was embarrassed because I did not even realize I was sniffing and snorting all the time.

We tested for Candida and food sensitivity using ELISA food sensitivity testing, which tests for delayed food sensitivities. I was sensitive to 38 of the 102 foods we tested. I was also loaded with Candida albicans, which is yeast commonly found in the digestive tract. It does not belong in the sinuses.

Mayo Clinic published a study that found this yeast in the sinuses of many people with chronic sinusitis. Unfortunately, the numbers of yeast grow every time one takes an antibiotic, eats a high-sugar meal, or takes hormones or birth control pills. The yeast then cause inflammation and blockage of the sinus drain passages, then bacterial infections start again. The perceived need for more antibiotics keeps the vicious cycle going along with a downward spiral in general levels of health.

The yeast/fungus can cause two problems:

1. We can become allergic to them. This causes an increase in the general allergen load. Because of the yeast allergy, the foods that

contain yeast and mold, like bread, cheese, mushrooms, and alcohol drinks, are often culprits. Diets high in sugar tend to feed yeast, so sugars and starchy foods add to the problem.

2. The yeast and fungus give off by-products as part of their metabolism. These wastes can be toxic, causing fibromyalgia, headaches, fatigue, joint pain, abdominal pain, and much more.

To properly treat this chronic sinusitis, the addition of a probiotic is a must. Probiotics are good bacteria that are naturally found in our body, sinuses, digestive tract, and vagina. They normally help keep the yeast in check, but antibiotics, steroids, and chlorinated water kill these good bugs. Use of these medications often puts the good bacteria in the sinus out of balance, letting the yeast grow wildly. Probiotics, usually acidophilus, should be taken orally two to four billion units per day. For chronic sinusitis, it is beneficial to put some probiotic in a saline nasal spray and squirt it up the nose four or five times per day.

Within six months, my snotty nose was much better. I only had post nasal drainage if I cheated with dairy products. As my body's sensitivity decreased, I was able to add most of the other foods to which I was sensitive back into my diet on a limited basis I have not had to take an antibiotic in over 15 years. What an amazing change.

So keep in mind, a sinus infection might be caused by an allergy. The yeast Candida albicans could be contributing to the problem. If you take antibiotics or steroids to treat the sinus infection, those medications will destroy the good, healthy flora in your system, which you should restore with some probiotics.

Be clear on this. You can solve this problem—and more. The bonus was that I eliminated 30 pounds of belly fat during that six months as well as feeling much, much better.

Sweet Death

To maintain a good healthy terrain within your body, you need carbohydrates. These are sugar and starches. Normally, these carbohydrates are burned for energy in our cells when our muscle is working. We can manufacture the carbohydrates that are essential for our survival; we do not need them in our diet. A small intake of carbohydrates is healthy for us. However, because these foods have a pleasing taste, we often eat much more of them than is healthy.

In 2004, Dr. Hugo Rodier, MD, published a book titled *Sweet Death*. In it, he explained quite clearly the dramatic effects of sugar. He also explains how Dr. John Yudkin, PhD, in the 1960s, was the first biochemist to write about the dangers of sugars.

There are many different kinds of sugars available to us. We need certain sugars to be healthy but certain kinds in large amounts are definitely hazardous to our health. Table sugar, sucrose, is made up of glucose and fructose.

Dr. Yudkin found that it was the fructose that was harmful. It causes increased blood levels of cholesterol, triglycerides, uric acid, insulin, and cortisol, all of which are associated with an increased risk of heart disease, strokes, and other degenerative diseases. It also raises blood pressure and increases the fragility of blood platelet cells, increasing risks of clots that can cause strokes and heart attacks.

Fructose in its natural form is found in fruit. In this form, it is not dangerous because the fruit contains fiber that slows down the absorption and enzymes that help break it down into small usable units.

The dangerous fructose comes from separation of the fructose from the food and heating it, destroying the enzymes. High fructose corn syrup (HFCS), which is a sweetener made from corn, is the most common. Sixteen billion pounds of this is manufactured each year, and it is added to just about all processed foods. Soft drinks have up to 12 teaspoons per 12 ounce can. Catsup has one teaspoon per tablespoon. And fruit juices are loaded. Also be aware that agave nectar, made from the starchy part of yucca roots, actually has higher fructose content than HFCS. Yet, it is often marketed in health food stores as a healthy alternative to table sugar.

Glucose can be used immediately for energy, but fructose must be first processed by the liver. In the liver, it is often converted to fat. Fructose gets priority in our system. This means that as long as there is processed fructose in our body, it must be handled first and other sugars that we ingest during that time period cannot be broken down until the fructose is all managed. As a result, we are often nutritionally starved and hungry even though the body has plenty of stored nutrients, in the form of glycogen and fat, just waiting to be used.

So, let's say you have a meal of a hamburger, French fries, and a Coke. The fructose from the soft drink must be processed first. Maybe it takes one to two hours for the liver to process all of the fructose, depending on how much you drank. During that time, the digestive mechanism is tied up and the glucose from the fries and the bread cannot be used, so it gets stored, first as glycogen and triglycerides then as fat. Maybe this is part of the reason we have so many over-weight issues in America.

If you want to live long and be healthy, it is imperative that you read labels and stop eating and drinking high fructose corn syrup. Go back to simply eating meat, vegetables, and fruit. Get rid of processed food. You will be able to eat all you desire and not be artificially starved. This is one great way that you can put your health in your own hands.

Diabetes

An increasing number of Americans are developing diabetes. People in many developing countries, like Japan, who are eating a more Western diet, are also experiencing a much higher rate of diabetes.

There are two forms of this disease:

- *Type 1* diabetes is a condition where the pancreas cannot produce enough insulin for the demand of the sugar load. In other words, if the body weight is too high or the intake of carbohydrates sugar and starch is too high for the amount of insulin that can be produced, the amount of sugar in the blood will go up. If the amount of sugar gets too high, serious effects can occur, including coma and death, although this is rare today. Most type 1 diabetics use insulin shots to replace the insulin that they cannot make.
- *Type 2* diabetes is a condition in which there is plenty of insulin; in most cases, too much insulin, but the cell membranes are defective and sugar cannot be transported into the cells where it can be used for energy.

The cell membranes have a very complicated mechanism of transporting sugar into the cells. When sugars and starches are eaten, they are broken down by enzymes (amylase) to glucose. This is absorbed into the blood. When the blood sugar goes up, the pancreas increases insulin production. The insulin then attaches to an insulin receptor on the surface of the cell, which acts like a docking station. This signals glucose transport pumps to be inserted into the cell membrane. These pumps then carry the glucose into the cell, thus reducing the amount of sugar in the blood and providing glucose for energy inside the cells. If the sugar load is too high or too fast, a very high amount of insulin is produced. This high insulin damages the insulin receptors, causing the glucose transport pumps to be reduced instead of increased. This leads to even higher levels of sugar that, in turn, leads to more inflammation and more damage to the receptors and pumps.

> **Case Study:** A few years ago, I had a 15-year-old female patient who weighed about 170 pounds. As part of working on her weight concerns, we did some blood tests. Included in that was an insulin level, which should be below 17. Her insulin level was 195, yet the amount of sugar in her blood was normal. This means she was pre-diabetic and her liver and pancreas were constantly compensating to keep the blood sugar in its normal range. Eventually, she will be unable to adjust, and she will become a full diabetic with uncontrolled blood sugars.

In an attempt to get rid of some sugar from the blood, our body does some interesting things.

- We convert sugar to triglycerides, which are three sugar molecules tied to a fat molecule. This is then stored as fat instead of being used for energy.
- We make some sugar into sorbitol, which is an alcohol that has anesthetic properties. But this can damage nerves, causing peripheral neuropathy, which is a burning pain and numbness in feet and legs.
- We dump sugar into the body fluids of sweat and urine, which causes more bladder and prostate infections as well as rashes and yeast infections. The high sugar causes more inflammation in the artery walls and plaque to build up.

Constant high blood sugar causes fat to be deposited in the omentum in the abdomen. The enzyme aromatase, produced by this fat, converts testosterone to estrogen, which leads to hormone imbalances and dysfunction.

Reducing sugar surges is the most important thing we can do to prevent type 2 diabetes. Eating small portions of high sugar foods and eating protein with high sugar foods slows down the absorption of sugar so there is no high sugar spike. This way, all the sugar ingested can be properly managed without getting the spikes in glucose that lead to all the damage.

Reducing weight and body mass so your body mass index (BMI) is below 25 is very beneficial. Herbal supplements that include chromium, vanadium, gymnema, nopal, and banaba leaf are all highly effective at reducing the insulin resistance. But this will only work long term if it is combined with portion control and weight control. The same is true for prescription medications. Using the glycemic index, which I describe in the next few pages, to help with food selection makes great sense.

Glycemic index

If you watch television at all, you will have seen advertisements for weight loss programs. They mention the glycemic index (GI). This is a system created to measure the relative amount of sugar in all foods, compared to glucose, which is the standard. Here are a few examples:

- The standard is pure glucose, which has a GI of 100.
- Table sugar is sucrose, which has a GI of about 70.
- Xylitol and stevia, which are natural sugar substitutes, have a GI of about 7.

Occasional high glycemic food is not a problem. However, when we do this daily, a series of complicated chemical and hormonal reactions occur in our bodies. The outcome is that energy from food gets stored as fat rather than being used for energy and vitality. We begin to increase weight, waist size, and risks for all sorts of serious health problems.

The simplest way to counteract this is to reduce the high glycemic foods, both in amount and frequency. But some people are so addicted to these foods that they find this very hard to do. Mixing the high glycemic food with low glycemic foods and fiber slows down the absorption of sugar. This will reduce the whole cascade of harmful risks that occur with the high GI foods by themselves.

Look, for example, at the peanut butter and jelly (PB&J) sandwich. The jelly and the white bread are high GI foods (GI around 70). The peanut butter is high in fat and protein and has a low GI. So PB&J on whole grain or Ezekiel bread has a much lower combined glycemic index. It is more likely to be absorbed more slowly into the system and therefore used by the body for energy than to be stored as fat.

This is why breakfast should contain protein, fats, and fiber as well as carbohydrates. An egg and whole grain or Ezekiel bread are better than cereal and milk. Lunches should contain protein and fats with some low GI carbohydrates. Dinner can be a small portion of meat and lots of vegetables but with no potatoes; one baked potato has a GI of 85, which is the same as eating six to eight teaspoons of table sugar. Snacks should be low glycemic foods. There are several good internet sites that give this information. Here is one that gives a lot: http://ultimatepaleoguide.com/glycemic-index.

As I was growing up, one of my uncles had a very large abdomen. We all thought it was funny how he could put his plate on his big belly to eat and did not have to use the table.

Now, many years later, I understand the seriousness of this condition, and unfortunately, he did die young. The formal medical term for this is visceral adipose tissue (VAT). It means fat deposited in the abdominal cavity. Hanging down over our internal organs is a thin fatty apron called the omentum. Its purpose is to protect our organs. It is within this omentum that the belly fat gets stored.

When we eat too much high glycemic food that has too much sugar and starch in it, we temporarily get high blood sugar. This causes too much insulin to be produced, creating a flurry of activity to get rid of the high blood sugar. Some of this extra sugar is converted to triglycerides, which can be converted into stored fat. In men, because of their higher testosterone, this fat goes to the omentum first and later to other parts of the body. In women, because of their higher estrogen, this fat goes to the buttocks and thighs first and then to the abdomen.

The worst part of this VAT accumulation is that it becomes an organ itself and it produces an enzyme called aromatase, which converts testosterone into estrogen. When men have increasing estrogen, they have a bunch of unwanted body changes. The prostate enlarges, causing urination problems and increasing numbers on the prostate-specific antigen (PSA) test. Sex drive and performance decreases. Breast enlargement and loss of muscle strength can occur. In women, estrogen dominance develops with all its weight control, emotional, and menstrual problems.

In both men and women, the next unwanted developments are high blood pressure, high cholesterol, and blood vessel diseases. So watch the waist. Ideal measurement, measured at the navel, is less than 40 inches for men and less than 32 inches for women. This will become the standard for monitoring risk in the future.

So the glycemic index, combined with portion control, becomes a great tool to reverse this whole process of unwanted fat deposition as well as all other health risks.

Syndrome X or metabolic syndrome

Syndrome X, also called metabolic syndrome, is a collection of symptoms and physical changes in the body that has been associated with a high number of deaths from blood vessel and heart disease.

The four main features are: non-insulin dependent diabetes (NIDDM), high blood pressure (hypertension), high cholesterol (hyperlipidemia), and increased body weight carried mostly in the abdomen and known as visceral abdominal obesity or the beer belly.

Non-insulin dependent diabetes is caused by insulin resistance. This means that high sugar loads in the diet cause the insulin receptors on the cell membranes to be damaged. When these do not work well, sugar cannot be removed from the blood and put into the cells for use as energy. As a result, the body makes more insulin to compensate for the high sugar. The insulin, already much higher than it should be, then causes inflammation of the blood vessel walls. In a response to this inflammation, LDL cholesterol increases, especially the small dense forms of LDL. These molecules of LDL are so small that they can get between the cells that line the arteries and underneath the epithelial cells. This causes more damage, leading to the buildup of plaque and the formation of blood clots and setting us up for heart disease and strokes.

In order to get rid of some of the sugar, triglycerides are formed of three sugar molecules attached to a fat molecule. The excessive triglycerides also cause damage and consequently more plaque to form. The excess sugars, because they cannot be burned for energy, are converted to fats and stored in the liver and in the abdomen causing the beer belly. The increased size of the abdomen causes the stomach to be pushed up leading to a hiatal hernia and gastro esophageal reflux disease (GERD) with its symptoms of acid reflux and heartburn that I described earlier. Because the sugars cannot be burned for energy, the brain detects starvation and kicks in the appetite, causing greater intake of sugars, adding more and more to the problem.

So you can see excess intake of sugar leads to all these conditions that the traditional medical community calls diseases. Reduce your sugar intake, and the symptoms go away.

The solution to syndrome X is to dramatically reduce the intake of glucose. Most carbohydrates, which are sugars and starches, break down to glucose. The glycemic index has been created to give us an idea of the relative amount of glucose in any food.

Xylitol is a good natural sugar substitute. It is a five-carbon sugar alcohol. The common sugars we use and all starches are composed of six carbon atoms. Xylitol occurs naturally in many plants. It has the sweetness of sucrose, which is table sugar, but 40 percent fewer calories and none of the insulin-release effects of refined sugars. The glycemic index of xylitol is 7, compared to table sugar of 65. Xylitol can reduce appetite. It can eliminate dental cavities. It can reduce staph infections (MRSA) by reducing the sugar content of sweat, therefore reducing the food supply to those bad bugs that can cause pimples, boils, and abscesses. And it can suppress appetite and reverse the spiral of insulin resistance.

One caution: xylitol can cause severe low blood sugar in dogs and is sometimes fatal. So do not feed xylitol-sweetened snacks to the family dog.

The details and benefits of this remarkable little product are detailed in a book *Sweet Death* by Dr. Hugo Rodier. It is important to understand that artificial sweeteners like NutraSweet, which is the brand name product for aspartame, and Splenda, the brand name product for sucralose, are very unhealthy. Most people do not realize that about one hour after using Splenda or NutraSweet, they will experience an increased appetite. This tends to aggravate the problem of weight control, and most people using these will gain an average of ten pounds per year.

If you have syndrome X or are addicted to sugar, try stevia or the xylitol yourself and see what results you get.

What is the most important lesson of syndrome X? Prevent it. Reduce the high sugar, high starch, and high glycemic foods from your diet now. That will avoid all those other issues later.

High cholesterol is not a disease

For the last 30 years, we have heard lots of things about cholesterol—mostly, how bad it is. Actually, cholesterol is very important to make hormones and nerve coverings, repair damaged arteries, and many other body functions.

Back in the old days of 30 to 40 years ago, we recommended very strict low-fat and low-cholesterol diets. And many times when people did that, the cholesterol would actually go up. That is because most of our cholesterol is actually manufactured by our own liver. In the absence of dietary cholesterol, the body simply made more.

Traditional medicine is really pushing medications that lower cholesterol, generically called statins, and constantly lowering the recommended limits. It is important to understand that the underlying problem is inflammation.

Before going into the role of inflammation, I need to explain two terms used in regard to cholesterol levels, as measured by laboratory blood tests. These are LDL and HDL.

LDL stands for low density lipoprotein. Lipoproteins are molecules made up of fat and protein. There are seven different kinds of LDL cholesterol, and they have many uses in the body. The difference in these seven sub-fractions has to do with their size and density. Think of a grapefruit, an apple, and an acorn. Each of these has a different size and density or hardness. LDL cholesterol is a carrier molecule, like a truck that carries freight. It circulates through our arteries, doing its job of carrying fats to all parts of the body where the fat is used for fuel, raw materials, and structural elements.

Our arteries have a tough outer layer, a muscle layer, and an inner lining called epithelium. That inner lining of our arteries is like a tightly woven cloth. The small, dense LDL particles are so small that they can get through the openings in the "cloth mesh." Once underneath the epithelial cells, these small, dense LDL particles create inflammation, acting like a sliver under the skin in your finger. This occurrence is the beginning of plaque buildup. This, then, is the basis of all arterial blood vessel disease, heart disease, and stroke.

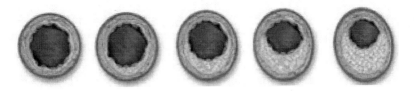

The drawing shows progression of plaque buildup, which is caused by the small dense sub-fraction of LDL cholesterol getting under the lining inside the artery walls. The plaque is represented by the whitish substance and blood inside the artery being the darker substance.

The letters HDL stand for high density lipoproteins. There are five kinds of HDL cholesterol. One of them, type 2a, is harmful. The rest function as artery cleaners. The number of HDL particles in your body increases with exercise. However, the amount and type of HDL particles are determined by the amount and type of exercise: anaerobic or aerobic.

Did you know you could exercise too much? Yes. Who would have thought that? How do you know what kind of exercise is good? I will detail that when I discuss exercise later on.

The type of LDL and HDL cholesterol that we produce is determined by what we eat, what kind of exercise we get, and by our Apo E Gene. We must think of food as fuel—it still can be tasty—instead of as entertainment. Elimination of toxins will decrease the production of small dense LDL, of the acorn size. Therefore, you will have less inflammation and less plaque.

An Ion Mobility Diagnostic Test and an Apo E Gene test from Berkley Heart Lab (now Quest Diagnostics) can determine how many of each of the seven sizes of LDL particles and the five kinds of HDL molecules are present in your blood.

You will notice heart disease rates are no lower now than they were 30 years ago. We need to reduce the inflammation and damage. Then the cholesterol will take care of itself, without medications. IgG Food Sensitivity, the Eat Right for Your Blood Type diet, and the Apo E Gene diet have worked very well for many people by reducing their intake of inflammatory food. Reducing smoking, excess alcohol, coffee, air pollution, chlorinated water, trans fats, microwave cooking, food additives, stress, and the amount of food consumed all significantly reduce inflammation. Drinking adequate amounts of water is very important; chronic dehydration causes a lot of damage.

Remember, reduce the inflammation, drink lots of water, and the cholesterol will take care of itself. Experiment with this over the next three to six months.

Cholesterol-lowering medications: Helpful or harmful?

On November 10, 2009, I heard on the news about a new study that showed taking the prescription drug Crestor produced nearly a 50 percent reduction in heart attacks and strokes in people with high C-reactive protein (CRP) but with normal or low cholesterol levels. The CRP is a blood test that has been used for years to determine the amount of inflammation in the arteries.

So I went to the internet, and, yes, there it was: a study of almost 18,000 people who had low or normal cholesterol were given this drug and it showed significant reduction in heart attacks and strokes. The key thing was that these people had an elevated CRP.

Now, before you run out and ask your doctor for a prescription for Crestor, here is the rest of the story:

- The manufacturer of Crestor paid for the study.
- The inventor of the CRP test, which cost about $80, was in charge of the study.
- The people in the study already had a very low heart attack and stroke risk of less than 13 out of 1,000.
- The people in the study had to have a healthy cholesterol level of less than 130 to get into the program.
- People who took Crestor had an increase in diabetes. (See www. diabetesupdate.blogspot.com)
- The number of people diagnosed with cancer during the study was 612. Is that significant?
- There were actually more fatal heart attacks in the Crestor group compared to the placebo group: nine compared to six. What does that mean?
- The cost of the drug is about $1,200.00 per year per patient.

- The study was two years long, and no one knows the effects of taking Crestor for 20 years.
- In 2011, the sale of statin drugs totaled $34 billion.
- The effects of the study are expected to boost sales of Crestor by $500 million.

Most of us are smart enough to see that this study is just an infomercial to promote sales of the drug and the test. We know to keep the advertised results in perspective.

Inflammation is the most important factor in the production of damage and blockage in our arteries. But, instead of taking a pill to reduce the cholesterol, why not do something natural to reduce the cause of the inflammation?

We also know we are responsible for causing most of our own health problems, either through poor nutrition, lack of exercise, or taking pills we don't need or want. There are over 900 published studies that show the harmful side effects of the cholesterol-lowering medications. In my opinion, highly sensitive people should not take these drugs and should turn to natural health practices instead. It is important to understand that there is no magic pill to help us live longer in perfect health; we have to put our health into our own hands.

Is my thyroid normal?

This is a question that every health care provider has heard many times. Most of the time, the question comes from patients who are experiencing fatigue or having weight concerns. Usually a lab test is done and the results are normal. Interestingly, the patients are often disappointed and sometimes a little angry.

There are some people who have thyroid resistance. Not really recognized by the traditional medical establishment, this is a condition in which the patient has adequate thyroid hormone but the body cannot use it properly. It is probable that this thyroid resistance is related to chlorine and fluoride from city water that blocks the iodine receptor sites on the cells.

Dr. Broda Barnes, MD, in his book *Hypothyroidism*, showed 40 years of research that supports the basal body temperature as a valid way of measuring the effects of thyroid activity. Motion and muscular activity produce heat, so the basal temperature is taken in the morning for ten minutes, under the arm, before getting out of bed. This should be done for four days. Women should take their temperatures for two days during their menstrual cycle and for two days off their menstrual cycle. The normal range for basal body temperature is 97.8 to 98.2 degrees. If the temperatures are below 96.0 degrees or above 99.5 degrees, there is a good chance the thyroid is not working correctly.

Avoid chlorine, bromine, and fluoride because these are in the halogen chemical family, the same as iodine, and they can interfere with the iodine receptors found on cell membranes.

Herbal Thyroid Activator, an herbal combination made by NSP, Kelp, Dulse, herbal Iodine, and other supplements can be taken to improve thyroid activity. Many times, these supplements will resolve the fatigue and other concerns. If they do not, further thyroid tests to check for antibodies and other more sophisticated abnormalities can be done.

Homeopathic Thyroidinum 6X has been shown to help "restart" an underactive thyroid. Application of the essential oil blend Valor over the thyroid has also proven to be very helpful.

Low dose medicine trials sometimes are used as both diagnosis and treatment, but most health care providers are reluctant to do this.

Vertigo

Vertigo is a nasty condition that bothers many people. The symptom of spinning dizziness might be mild or so severe that a person cannot stand up. Nausea is often a part of it. It is usually caused by an imbalance in the inner ear related to trauma, viral infection, poor circulation, or diet.

Each ear has three parts: the outer or external ear, the middle ear, and the inner ear.

The outer or external ear consists of the pinna, which is the part you feel when you touch your ear, and the ear canal where wax sometimes accumulates.

The external ear and the middle ear are separated by the tympanic membrane or ear drum. The middle ear has three small bones, called ossicles, the smallest bones in the human body, that transmit vibration from the tympanic membrane to the hearing apparatus of the inner ear.

The inner ear has two parts: the cochlea, which is the hearing apparatus, and the balance mechanism. The balance mechanism in each inner ear contains three semi-circular canals. One is positioned horizontally; one is vertical from left to right; and one is vertical from front to back. This positioning of one canal on each of these planes allows us to stay oriented and aware of our position in space, to know which end is up.

Each canal in the inner ear is a hollow tube, shaped like a ring and filled with fluid. Near the bottom is a wide spot with a layer of hair cells, much like bristles on a flat hair brush. Balanced on these hair cells is a small stone, called an otolith.

When we move, the fluid pushes the otolith to one side and the brain interprets the movement of the hair cells as motion. Sometimes, the otolith gets stuck or the fluid begins to move on its own, and we have a sensation of spinning. This is the physical cause behind vertigo.

Dietary causes of vertigo are too much alcohol, salt, and salty food like ham, bacon, chips, popcorn, and so on. Not enough water intake can also be a factor. We always see a lot of vertigo around the holidays when people eat salty food, drink too much alcohol, and do not drink enough water.

Every day, we should drink approximately an amount of pure water that, measured in ounces, is equal to 1/3 to 1/2 our body weight in pounds, up to 100 ounces. For example, if you weigh 200 pounds, the volume of water you consume should be 60 to 100 ounces. A person who weighs a petite 110 pounds should consume 30 to 50 ounces. Pop and coffee do not count and actually might make the problem of dehydration worse. Please understand that these are guidelines and your individual needs may vary. Do not get hung up on exact amounts.

When the inner ear is the cause of the problem, you can use Epley's Maneuvers to recalibrate the otoliths in the semi-circular canals. To see a video of this, go to the internet at www.youtube.com, and then enter Epley's Maneuver for Vertigo. There will be several clips to show you what to do, but here is a verbal description of the maneuver.

1. Start by lying on your back, then turn your head as far to the affected side as comfortable and hold that position for 20 to 30 seconds.

2. Next, turn your head to the other side and hold that position for 20 to 30 seconds.

3. Next, roll onto your side, keeping your head in the same position with respect to your body so that you will be looking toward the floor. Hold that position for 20 to 30 seconds.

4. Then sit up slowly, again keep the head turned to the unaffected side.

If both ears are affected, repeat this process, starting with other side the second time. If you are not sure which side is affected most, just do the procedure in both directions.

This simple technique, along with salt restriction and good hydration, will successfully manage about 80 percent of the cases of vertigo. Homeopathic Cocculus 30C can be added, one pellet every 30 to 60 minutes, to assist with moderate cases. Prescription Antivert, Phenergan for nausea, and oral steroids might be needed for more severe cases.

Tinnitus or ringing in the ears

This is an aggravating condition of the inner ear characterized by a variety of noises in the ears. The cause is unknown but seems to be associated with exposure to excess noise, sudden loud noises, trauma, infection, and sometimes calcification in the inner ear.

When I worked with Dr. Born at the Born Clinic in Grand Rapids, Michigan, we saw many cases of tinnitus clear after intravenous chelation treatment. I have used herbal Hydrangea, one capsule three times per day, and homeopathic Calcerea Carbonicum 6C once per day with good results if the problem happens to be due to calcium build up in the inner ear or around the openings in the bones for the nerves and blood vessels that supply the inner ear. We also use homeopathic Cinchona Sulphuricum 6C or 12C once per day with fair results. A two or three month trial is inexpensive and not likely to be harmful.

Hair

In the animal world, hair and feathers are used to attract mates and partners. It is not so different with human animals who, socially, view hair is a very important part of our body. Every day, I hear complaints about hair. Too-much. Too much in the wrong places. Too little in the right places. Too curly. Too straight. The wrong color. And on and on.

Healthy hair requires certain conditions. Hair is extruded up from the hair follicle. In the follicle, all the ingredients to make the hair shaft are assembled, much like the process of toothpaste being extruded out through the top of the tube. If the correct ingredients are not brought to the hair follicle by the blood vessels, normal hair cannot be produced. Good blood flow is needed. Protein, amino acids, fats, oils, carbohydrates, minerals, and vitamins are all needed to create this amazing filament we know as hair.

The little factories that make the fibers of hair are affected by hormones. Thyroid, testosterone, progesterone, estrogen, and many more hormones are like a labor force that may call a strike. They are affected by stress. So stress management is a must for balanced hormones—and healthy hair. If needed, get a hormone blood or saliva test and take natural bio-identical hormone replacement if the hormones are out of balance.

Existing hair can be damaged and broken by physical trauma like hair twirling or wearing caps and hair bands. Hair shafts can also be damaged by the chemicals in hair care products.

Genetics definitely play a role. So in order to have great healthy hair on your head, be sure to pick the right parents. Oh, well, too late now. So, even if you did not pick parents with healthy hair, we know from the study of epigenetics that keeping a healthy terrain around the hair follicle might overcome some of the effects of the bad hair genetics.

Elimination of toxins in the blood is a must. Toxins like tobacco, alcohol, coffee, pop, and inflammatory foods have a huge negative impact on our hair. Other things like lead, mercury, cadmium, trans fats, chemicals from shampoo, perm solutions, and hair coloring can hurt the hair as it is being made. Trans fats, which include vegetable oil, deep fried food, and animal fat, especially feed-lot beef and pork, are damaging to hair. So are excessively washing the hair; lack of brushing, which brings scalp oil into the hair shaft; excess heat, such as from a hot hair dryer; and too much direct sunshine, which can fry the hair.

Nutrients, amino acids, healthy oils, and sugars are needed to enrich hair. Hair has to have oils like olive oil and flax seed oil as well as fiber and complex carbohydrates from vegetables. Chondroitin, glucosamine, and methylsulfonylmethane (MSM), which we get from animal cartilage and gelatin, are essential for healthy hair, skin, and nails. We like a product from NSP, Hair, Skin, and Nails (HSN). Silica, silver, tin, other trace minerals, and vitamins E and D3 are a must.

Your hair is a good barometer of the health of the rest of your body. If it is unhealthy, thin, weak, and wispy, maybe other things are not so healthy either. Look to your hair for guidance as you make some changes.

Skin

Our skin is actually the largest organ of our body. It has many functions besides presenting our good looks. One function is physical protection. It is our first line of defense against chemical and microbial invasion. The skin is made up of about 15 layers of dead cells held together by a fatty cement. Viruses need live cells to reproduce, so our skin is our first level of anti-viral protection. The oils in the skin help protect us from toxins and chemicals that might injure our more internal parts. The skin makes melanin, which is a black pigment that protects us from sun damage. The sweat glands help us stay cool. Little muscles in the skin, known as erector pili muscles, cause goose bumps that help regulate heat. Tiny ring muscles in the arteries also open and close to help control heating and cooling.

The skin oil glands and sweat glands are part of our routes of elimination; the others are kidneys/bladder, colon, lungs, as I've written about earlier. If the normal routes of elimination for wastes are not working well, we might start to dump wastes through the skin, which results in bad body odor and acne.

Healthy hair, skin, and nails require certain nutritional ingredients to be able to manufacture the collagen, oils, and other components that make up the skin. Adequate water is a must for healthy skin. Chondroitin, glucosamine, and methylsulfonylmethane (MSM) are compounds that our body uses to make healthy skin, hair, and nails. Plant oils that contain omega-6 and omega-9 fatty acids, like olive oil, coconut oil, and flaxseed oil, are very useful for making good, healthy skin oil. If we do not have enough of these in our diet, we will get sebaceous cysts, acne, eczema, psoriasis, dry skin, cradle cap, and weak hair. This happens because the oil begins to turn into a wax that plugs the pores and causes white heads and black heads. Some people should avoid perfumes and fragrant lotions because they are often toxic to the skin. For sensitive people, we recommend essential oil by Young Living as an alternative to perfumes and fragrances.

Recommendations for healthy hair, skin, and nails are:

- 2 oz. of olive oil daily;
- 2000 mg of fish oil or flaxseed oil per day;
- 400 IUs of vitamin E, use d alpha Tocopherol, not l or dl forms;
- 1200 to 1500 mg of chondroitin twice per day, but men should avoid this if the PSA is elevated or prostate cancer is present;
- 1200 to 1500 mg of glucosamine twice per day;
- 500 mg of MSM twice per day;
- 40 to 60 oz. of water per day;
- frequent skin brushing, massage, and hot sweaty exercise;
- a colon cleanse twice a year;
- a liver cleanse two to four times per year; and
- adequate daily intake of pure water.

Do some or all of these, and you will look, smell, and feel great.

Eczema and psoriasis

Eczema and psoriasis are two very aggravating skin conditions. Huge amounts of money are spent every year by patients trying to get these two under control.

Eczema usually has red scaly patches that sometime weep a yellow fluid that can lead to a yellow crust. Psoriasis usually has red scaly patches. The crusty scale is usually silvery white. These might itch and be irritating. They often occur on the elbows and knees.

Some people believe the cause of psoriasis is a fungal infection, and allergies are definitely a component of eczema. Traditional treatment is usually topical steroid creams. Sunlight is always helpful and often ultraviolet light treatments are used. Thirty minutes of sunshine every day, before 10 am and after 2 pm, are vital for controlling these two conditions.

Both of these conditions are nicely treatable using natural methods because they are internal problems.

In addition to the recommendations for healthy skin in the last section, the following nutritional approaches suggest diets that are low in sugar and acidity are very helpful; this means reduce red meat, pop, sugar, tomatoes, and oranges. Eating green leafy vegetables is a must. I feel that people with eczema should strictly avoid all dairy products. Drinking an adequate amount of water is extremely important.

Homeopathic remedies must be individualized to each person with these conditions. In general, Graphites 6C, Petroleum 6C, and Sulphur 6C are good remedies to start with, but usually others and higher doses will be needed, depending on the person.

Migraine headaches

Many people suffer from head pain. I have had two migraines in my life, and they were truly incapacitating.

The physical mechanics of phase one of migraine headaches are as follows:

- Something causes a cluster of blood vessels in a part of the brain to contract; this is called vasoconstriction. This might last for five to sixty minutes.
- During the period of vasoconstriction, many people will experience something called an aura, which is a warning that phase two is coming.

The aura symptoms can be very frightening, especially the first time they occur. They include nausea; photosensitivity in which light bothers the eyes; sensitivity to noise; smelling odors that are not present; strange tastes in the mouth; flashes of light, wavy lines, blind spots, blindness in half of the visual field or in one eye; weakness in part of the body; creepy feelings in one part of the body; garbled speech; and more.

Phase two of the migraine involves a change in the blood vessels from constriction to dilation. When the constricted blood vessels begin to dilate or enlarge, that part of the brain becomes engorged with blood. The pressure that was then applied on the brain coverings and surrounding tissues causes the pain of the migraine. There is some new evidence now that dilation of the blood vessels of the scalp could play a bigger role in the head pain than dilation of the brain blood vessels.

The aura can occur without pain, which is a condition called a silent migraine. And the pain can occur without the aura. Abdominal migraines can occur, causing the phase two pain to be in the abdomen instead of the head.

Natural treatment focuses around what causes the initial constriction of the blood vessels. We believe that the cause of most of these headaches is a chemical trigger that comes from foods or toxins. The cumulative effect of food additives, preservatives, pesticides, herbicides, hormones, etc. as well as toxins in our air and water undoubtedly have some effect on the blood vessels and nerves of a genetically susceptible person. The offending trigger causes the cascade of events that lead to pain.

We think the first step toward perfect health is a colon cleanse. When I first heard this, I laughed. How could the bowel be connected to headaches? But they are. A colon cleanse heals the bowel lining so wastes and toxins in our food go down the toilet and are not re-absorbed into our blood. And healthy blood, of course, is necessary for proper brain function. However, when a person is weak and debilitated, cleanses should be avoided or used under the guidance of a professional who is knowledgeable in this area.

Exercise is very important. Muscular activity moves waste by-products from our cells through the lymphatic system to our routes of elimination and out of the body.

Food journals often identify triggers. Foods can affect us up to four days after we eat them. So, after a migraine, write down everything you have eaten for the previous four days. If you have recurring migraines, you might see a pattern emerge.

Proper hydration is a must to eliminate head pain. Chronic dehydration and electrolyte imbalance is a factor in most types of headache.

You can also follow the "eliminate, challenge, and observe" protocol for the following food groups: dairy, wheat, corn, eggs, and yeast. Eliminate one food group at a time for two weeks, then challenge by eating foods in that group for one day, then observe for four days. If no migraine is triggered, go to the next group. If you get a headache after the challenge step, you know that food group is part of the trigger. The trigger can be a component of the food or an additive if it is a processed food. Completely eliminate that group from your diet for three months and try it again.

Reactions can be related to the quantity of food consumed and can be a cumulative effect of several foods from a certain group. Look to foods and your digestive system for the answer to migraines.

There can be emotional and stress causes.

Stress is associated with what is called the fight-or-flight response in our body. When we sense danger, we are genetically programmed to respond to this danger by running to safety or fighting for our survival. Our pulse rate goes up. Blood pressure rises. Breathing rate increases. Blood sugar goes up. Muscles tense. Everything is preparing and getting ready to meet the challenge. The release of adrenalin causes vasoconstriction, part of the first phase of a migraine. So every time sensitive people get stressed, they are right on the verge of triggering a migraine.

Our body is designed to meet these fight-or-flight episodes and then recover. However, when our body is constantly bombarded by stressful events, we sometimes begin to break down our genetically weakest system.

Stress causes the damage to the system and becomes part of the trigger that starts the chemical cascade in our body that presents itself as a migraine. Stress is a natural, normal part of being human. We cannot really get away from it. So what do we do? We can learn to change how we respond to it.

In the traditional medical world, doctors prescribe medications that dampen our reaction to the stress triggers. In theory, this is good. But in the long run, it does not work very well because people tend to get addicted to the medications. They then have a new set of problems and stressors to deal with.

The best way to deal with stress is to learn to change how our body reacts to the fight-or-flight triggers. When we have learned this, our automatic response to the stressful trigger is not an increase in blood pressure and pulse but a calm, cool mind and body that can handle the situation without damaging the system.

Learning basic relaxation and meditation techniques is where we should begin. Many years ago, I learned a few simple things and since then have studied much more advanced techniques. We suggest starting with a relaxation class or a recording like the *Mind Coaching* CDs that I recorded and mentioned earlier in this book to calm the mind. Spend a little time each day practicing these mental training exercises in the morning before getting out of bed, after lunch in the afternoon, and just before going to sleep. Once per day is good; twice per day is very good; and three times per day is excellent.

The technique is as simple as sitting in a quiet, comfortable place where you will not be disturbed for 10 or 15 minutes. Then close your eyes and inhale a deep breath. As you exhale, consciously feel your body relax. Mentally imagine you are at an ideal place of relaxation. This could be a place you have been before or a completely imaginary place. Your brain cannot tell the difference between actually being there and vividly imagining that you are there. Then daydream in this pleasant state of mind, relaxing both body and mind.

Doing this regularly will replace stress chemistry with relaxation chemistry and will begin the repair process in your body. With practice, your emergency response will be calm and resourceful instead of fight-or-flight, and the frequency and intensity of the migraines will change and eventually disappear.

Head pain caused by muscle tension

Millions of people suffer from headaches, yet many millions more have never had a headache. Why? It is natural not to have head pain, so pain is telling us that something is wrong. It is telling us to look for the cause of the pain and fix it. It is important to know there is always a cause, a reason for every symptom.

The causes for headaches might be physical, mental, or emotional.

Physical causes include muscle tension, migraine headaches, sinus congestion, allergic reactions, head injury, and withdrawal from pain medication and stimulants.

> **Case Study:** WM was an elderly man who lived in an adult foster care home. He complained of head pain in the right posterior region of his head since bumping his head during a fall. He had had many tests and an MRI, all with negative results. But his scalp was so sensitive that even light touch or hair combing was very painful. I suggested homeopathic Hypericum 30C once per day for ten days and topical applications of Frankincense essential oil three or four times per day. By the time of his three week follow-up visit, he was pain free and has remained so.

Muscle tension in the head, face, and scalp is the result of tightening muscles, and it has many sources:

- Squinting from poor vision, ill-fitting or poorly corrected glasses
- Inflammation in the temporal mandibular joint (TMJ), which is the joint that hinges the jaw
- Degenerative arthritis from old injuries in the neck as the muscles there try to hold the neck from moving to reduce bone and joint pain
- Head and facial trauma, which can also leave trigger points that cause muscles to shorten
- Long, heavy hair or hair pulled too tightly into a pony tail
- Hats that are too tight
- Too much frowning or too much smiling

The pain from muscle tension has several causes. When a muscle is held too tightly:

- it cannot get proper blood flow, causing the capillaries to become pinched;
- waste products such as lactic acid and others cannot be removed by the lymphatic system, which needs motion to work;
- the tendons that attach muscle to the periosteum, the bone covering, gets stressed and will sometimes begin to lift off the bone; and
- the muscle contraction units, called myofibrils, might become damaged.

All these things can occur when there is not enough motion within a muscle. This leads to a "normal" reaction to injury called inflammation. This reaction to injury causes release of chemicals, called kinens, which our nerve sensors record as pain.

So, if the pain of a muscle tension headache has the above causes, it is clear that the solution is not in a pill but in movement and lengthening the affected muscles. Correcting the cause behind the muscle tightness is necessary. Get the glasses tuned up. Avoid the tight cap. Loosen the pony tail. Thin or cut and donate the heavy hair.

The pain of TMJ syndrome can be relieved by wearing a bite splint, which is a football player's mouth guard, at night. Before bed, apply one drop of the essential oil Lavender in front of each ear and apply some heat for ten minutes. Then open your mouth wide and massage from the lower ears up into your temples for four to five minutes. This will hurt at first but the technique will eventually stretch the muscles and eliminate the pain. You can do this stretch massage several times per day. Later, I will discuss how to release the emotional stress that causes one to clinch their teeth.

Stretching the head and neck muscles every morning or throughout the day will keep them loose and limber. Massage is an excellent way to stretch, loosen, and re-educate a muscle that has lost its memory for the neutral position. Acupuncture, myotherapy, trigger point release, chiropractic, yoga, and Reiki are all great methods to deal with muscle tension pain.

Remember, do not stop with the diagnosis; look for and find the cause behind it. In your search you must always ask, "Why?" Keep looking for the cause until you heal yourself.

Natural Treatments

Earlier in this book, I discussed the hierarchy of natural medicine treatment. We believe that nutrition is the first and most important part of natural treatment. Then there are herbs, supplements, tinctures, Bach Flower remedies, homeopathic remedies, essential oils, and energy medicine. All of it has a place. In this section, I will discuss some of the therapeutics in more detail.

Are you a temple or a party store?

Many of us have heard the statement that our body is the temple where our soul lives. A few weeks ago, Barb was giving a talk on nutrition. She asked this question of the audience: "Is your body a temple or a party store?" It struck me that this is a great analogy for where some of us are and where some of us would like to be in regard to our health. Now, if we add to that the concept of mind-body-spirit, we can create a great model for how to live.

If our body were a physical temple, what would it look like? It would be strong and muscular. The skin smooth and clear. The eyes bright and sparkling. The nose open and able to smell everything. The tongue clean and able to experience the full range of gustatory delights or tastes. (I just love that word, gustatory). The hearing sharp.

We would be able to breathe fully and run with ease. Our pounding heart would provide nourishment to all cells and tissues. Digestion and assimilation of nutrients would be flawless. The elimination of wastes through the skin, lungs, kidneys, and bowels would keep the body fresh and vibrant. The hands would be flexible with excellent fine motor skills. Feet and legs would carry us with poise and efficiency. Our back would be strong and supportive of all our physical activity. Daily exercise would be an enjoyable routine.

In other words, our body would be an efficient machine, doing everything we desire it to do.

If our mind were a mental temple, what would it look like? The memory would be sharp and clear. We would focus or daydream according to what we need at the time. We would be funny and enjoy a great laugh. Our thoughts would be peaceful and comfortable. We would see the good in everyone and every situation. We would know that everything happens for a reason and a purpose that serves us in some way, even if we do not understand it. We would hang out with joyful, loving people. We would use our minds to plan and create great things, and we would wallow in successful outcomes.

If our whole being were a spiritual temple, what would life be like? We would have a time of prayer, meditation, and contemplation. Unconditional love for everyone we meet would be automatic. Throughout the day, we would take time to marvel at the wonder and majesty of God's creation. We would read and study with the innocent, open mindedness of a child.

Now I want you to picture a party store that is brightly lit and inviting but is also filled with many things that we intuitively know are not healthy for us: alcohol, tobacco, pop, coffee, junk food, processed food with many additives and preservatives, and so on. Many stores are like this and they provide an important service for many people.

But some party stories are also dirty, grimy, and dimly lit. Maybe they sell pornography. Outside, some seedy characters are pushing drugs. The energy of this place is low and dark. The atmosphere is offensive.

These images are not intended to offend any of the great people who provide a clean, convenient shopping environment. But the analogy is intended to give you the idea that we all find ourselves somewhere on the teeter-totter between the temple and the party store. We are all exposed, either daily or at some time, to foods and materials that are not healthy for us. Sometimes, we take some of those unhealthy items into our body and our mind; sometimes they affect our spirit.

As you move back and forth, day by day, keep the model of the temple in your mind as your ideal. You will slowly be attracted to do those things that will bring you closer to that place where your soul does live in a temple.

Biological terrain

A few years ago, the oil spill in the Gulf of Mexico was spewing oil into the ocean, threatening marine life and disrupting the coastal habitat. Ecologists were going crazy, and we recalled pictures of the Alaskan spill in the 1980s with the oil-covered shoreline and many sea creatures dead.

At the time of the Gulf spill, there was a discussion on National Public Radio about an ecosystem in one of the coastal marshlands. In this area, crabs feed on snails that eat a certain species of grass. Everything is in balance and has been so for many, many years. With the oil approaching, there was a fear that the crabs would die and the snails would have no natural predators, then they would overfeed on the grass and the marsh would die within a short time. This would have a ripple effect on lots of other organisms and might even indirectly impact human lives.

This situation reminds me of the biological terrain in our bodies. Everything should be in balance. When we ingest some medicines like antibiotics, steroids (prednisone), birth control pills, or hormones, we can kill off the healthy normal flora in our intestines. These healthy bacteria, called probiotics, help with digestion and keep the population of bad bacteria and yeasts under control, just like the crabs, snails, and grasses all maintain a balance with each other. Coffee, pop, alcohol, high fructose corn syrup, sugar, and food additives can all have the same negative effect on the good bugs in the digestive system.

Yeasts are normal and necessary in our small intestine. They clean up undigested sugars, preventing them from entering the large intestine. But when we have no good bugs to keep the yeast in balance, they over-grow out of control. This causes some people to become allergic to yeast and mold in food and the air. It also causes a release of toxins that are waste by-products from the yeast into our system, causing chronic fatigue, fibromyalgia, irritable bowel syndrome, irritable bladder syndrome, memory loss, and a whole host of other unpleasant conditions.

The biological terrain of our digestive track is in a delicate balance. It can take small insults and compensate for some toxic stuff like the usual trash that washes up on the beaches. But when there is a massive insult, like the oil spill, it can have huge and devastating impacts on our body, just like the sea creatures and the marshlands.

Think about how good, natural, organic, healthy food keeps things in balance. Think about all the toxic stuff we put into our body that throws off the biological terrain. So let's not fool with Mother Nature. Keep things as pure and natural as possible.

Eating plan for achieving ideal body shape and size

There are a million ideas about diet and nutrition and about how we should eat. All of them promise great success and magic weight loss. Most of the time, however, these ideas are the stories of individuals who were very ill. Often, they found something that worked for them and then they spread the word, thinking that this should work for everyone.

We have found that a successful food plan must be personalized for every individual. We like to use the plan created by Dr. Peter D'Adamo in his book *Eat Right for Your Type*. This is one of the best books I have seen because it takes a holistic approach. If your blood type and the blood type of your parents are the same, then this program will be quite accurate for you. If the blood type of you and your parents do not match, then you will likely have characteristics of all the types involved.

We also use *The Apo E Gene Diet* or *The Perfect Gene Diet*, which are actually the same book by Pamela McDonald printed by different publishers. This is a breakthrough book that deals with the use of the Apo E Genotype information to select food and exercise. The testing can be expensive but this is the program I use to maintain my slender body mass index (BMI) of 22.

Over the next few months of working with one of these programs, you will figure out the best plan for yourself. Remember you're on a quest, a journey. You are an extremely complex being, and determining the best food plan for you to achieve an ideal waist and body size will be a fun project. Think of it as a process. Like a pregnancy, it takes some time and the correct things have to happen before the desired outcome is realized. And best of all, it will be worth it.

There are only three things for you to focus on. One is your eating schedule, second is your eating location, and the third is portion control. Do not jump into any fad diet or severe deprivation program at this time. Your mind needs to adjust to what you are planning and your body needs to be cleansed first.

You might need to adjust your current *eating schedule*. After your wake-up meditation, drink four ounces of hot water or hot lemon water (one half of a lemon squeezed into four ounces of hot water) or a four-ounce cup of hot green tea or Pau D'Arco herbal tea. This will be your signal to your body, especially your liver, to wake up and get moving. Next eat breakfast.

At mid-morning, have a small snack that must contain all three major food groups: fats, protein, and carbohydrates. Then have lunch, a mid-afternoon protein snack, and, finally, eat supper. Before bed, drink two ounces of warm water or a nighttime tonic. We will explain this and deal with the content of meals and snacks later. For now, just change your eating schedule if you are not currently eating this way. You are not a cow, so do your best not to graze. Eat only at these five times approximately every three hours.

Next, look at your *eating location*. This is a huge part of the behavior change needed to bring this quest to your ultimate outcome. Many of us eat in many locations: the car, bed, couch, bathroom, work station. To facilitate body changes, it is very important to think about and then implement changes to eat only in appropriate eating places that are designed for eating and intake of energy: the kitchen, dining room, lunch room, picnic table on the patio, a local restaurant, and so on. You have to go to the gas station to fill your car with fuel. It is the same with your body. It is best if you go to one of your eating places for meals and snacks.

Your body will respond, just like Pavlov's dogs,[3] to the triggers of going to the eating places. We function on a complex matrix of habits, programmed into us by our previous repetitive actions. When we eat in bed or on the couch all the time, these locations can trigger food urges. You want your body to prepare for eating only in your eating locations. If you have been eating in these non-eating locations, you have triggers to eat in these locations. Therefore, you should scramble things up a little by moving the furniture around and changing the location of things in your rooms.

Portion control is a key factor in management of your waist size. Rent, borrow, or purchase a copy of the movie *Super Size Me* by David Morrow. In this documentary, Morrow ate at McDonald's three times a day for one month. He gained 27 pounds and his cholesterol went from 180 to 240. This movie has many lessons, but our main focus, in regard to your eating plan, is the amount of food he ate during those 30 days—a tremendous amount of simple carbohydrates found in breads, potatoes, and waffles and high fructose corn syrup in pop and syrup.

---

3. In 1904, Russian scientist, Ivan Pavlov won the Nobel Prize in Physiology for his research in physiologic conditioning. He observed that when he fed his research dogs, they would drool profusely. The dogs were kept in a kennel. When the kennel door opened, a bell would ring. What he noticed and later studied was that after a while the dogs would drool when the bell rang, even if there was no food for them to eat.

Many of us belong to the Clean Your Plate Club. I still remember my father placing a sign near our table that contained an idea he got while in the US Army: "Take all you want, but eat all you take." When the authority figures in our lives condition us to do a certain behavior, we will often do that behavior repetitively for our whole lives. It is important not to be wasteful (or is it "waist full"). However, it is better for your body to break this habit if you have it. Program yourself to leave some small portion of food on your plate at every meal. This gradually overcomes the old habit of always cleaning your plate.

If you hold your palms together to make a small bowl, this is the size of your normal stomach, and you only have enough digestive enzymes available at any one time to break down and digest that amount of food. Hold your hands together in the shape of a bowl right now and look at them. Imagine that amount of food on your plate for your entire meal. You might feel like that is not enough. You might even feel a little panic. But as your mind changes, you will become comfortable with that smaller amount of food for your meals. Remember, you are changing to a new comfort zone.

Eat from a smaller plate. Recently, Barb and I were on a cruise. The food was buffet style with gigantic platters for plates. We would fill our platters—and you probably would too. We all have genetic memory of starvation. Where there is food and a container to hold it, we will naturally take as much as we can. So use a salad plate for your meals. That will help maintain the proper portions.

Do not place food on the table in serving dishes—except for major holiday meals. The food in the serving dishes is a great temptation to pick at and take second helpings after you have finished your portion of food. If you are the cook in the household, learn to prepare smaller portions of food for each meal. When dining in a restaurant, consider sharing your meal with your companion or ordering a half meal or a "senior portion," which is usually smaller.

Avoid pre-packaged food plans through which you buy a company's food or specially prepared meals. These plans will help you to eliminate weight as long as you eat the allotted amount of their pre-packaged food. But will you do that the rest of your life? Probably not. You must relearn to eat correctly, in your eating places and with only appropriate portions for your physical body's needs. The majority of the food you eat will be natural and prepared by you or a family member.

Virtual Gastric Band Hypnosis

In 2012, I discovered an amazing weight control program called Sheila Granger's Virtual Gastric Band Hypnosis. Here is what I wrote about it in January 2013:

Well, everyone, the holidays are finally over and we can get back to real life. But then there is our health. And some of us went way overboard and gained a bunch of weight with all the parties and celebrations since Thanksgiving Day.

But this is not the case with a group of people who have attended The Virtual Gastric Band Hypnosis program. In the months of November and December, over 20 people completed this program. All of them either eliminated weight or maintained their weight through this difficult time of the year. And all have a huge head start on the New Year.

This program teaches eating and food awareness. It is not a diet. You can eat anything you want. Because you feel full faster, you automatically eat less. If you reduce your food intake by 100 calories per day, in one year, you will eliminate ten pounds. The opposite is also true. This is how people gradually become bigger.

One of our graduates tells about going to the theater. Instead of eating a gigantic bucket of popcorn, using both hands to shovel it in, she bought a small bag. Eating just one kernel at a time and enjoying the taste of each bite, she ate only half the bag through the whole movie.

Another graduate writes that she eliminated 13 pounds in the first three weeks. A young man who started the first class, but never completed it because of work conflicts, has eliminated over 20 pounds in five weeks.

One woman tearfully writes, "My husband bought a necklace for me on Sweetest Day, but I couldn't wear it because it was too tight on my neck. After five weeks on this program, I can wear this necklace and it feels so good. Thank you!"

"I had to cut and sell a lot of firewood to pay for this program, but it was well worth it," one graduate told us.

What are you waiting for? If you join us now, by next year this time, you will be the size and shape that you desire to be. Just imagine that for a moment.

We do not focus on weight. We teach you to eat mindfully, enjoying every bite, being satisfied with those three small meals per day.

We all know what to do, but something holds us back and we just don't do it. What do you have to lose?

By January 2014, we have had about 75 graduates of this program. Many have returned for the free refresher available to people who have gone through the program. We do not keep statistics, but generally everyone is doing well, living healthier and smaller. You can participate in the program in person, individually or in a group, or by phone. See our website for more information: www.thehealingcenteroflakeview.com.

Breakfast

An interesting study in the Journal of Pediatrics in 2008 showed that eating breakfast had a significant impact on the weight of teenagers and adults. This study of 2,200 teenagers in the Minneapolis, Minnesota, area looked at their average body mass index (BMI).

The BMI is a measuring tool that compares weight-to-height ratios (weight in kilograms divided by height in meters squared). A BMI of 18 to 25 is considered healthy, anything over 25 is considered overweight, and over 30 is considered obese. BMI calculators can be found on the internet or at your doctor's office.

The study showed that teens who ate breakfast had a BMI of 21.7 on average and those who did not eat breakfast had a BMI of 23.4. These people were followed up five years later, and the study found that the pattern had stayed the same. Those who did not eat breakfast had considerably more weight-related health problems.

As many as 34 percent of teenagers do not eat breakfast.

In natural health, we recommend all meals and snacks should be balanced with fats, carbohydrates, and protein. A Pop-Tart and a Coke is not really the best breakfast. Eat about every three hours and think of food as fuel, not entertainment.

The word "breakfast" is actually a blend of two words: "break" and "fast" that tells us what that meal is all about—to break the overnight fast. At night, our digestive system, including the liver, is supposed to rest and recharge itself. Literally, to "break fast" means to start things up again for the new day. A cup of hot lemon or hot herbal tea, followed by a meal, is one of the best ways to start the day. Coffee, the choice of millions, is too acidic and does not really assist in the startup of all the enzyme systems that need to get going. If you must drink coffee, make it weak—you should be able to see through it—and limit it to one or two cups. Remember, it takes 400 mg of calcium to buffer or neutralize the acid in one cup of strong coffee. This is important to know if you are at risk for osteoporosis.

Have a lunch with meat or some form of protein in it. This will enable your body to digest all the protein by 8:00 pm. Then, you and your liver will be able to shut down for the night and rest.

If you eat a big meal with lots of meat for supper, the liver has to continue operations until past midnight and it gets very little down time. This often contributes to insomnia.

So, consider an experiment for three to four weeks. Have a good balanced breakfast, a high-protein lunch, and a light low-protein supper. See how you feel after a month or so. Things will most likely be much better.

Fasting for health

I wrote this just after I completed a four-day fast. Of course, this makes me an expert. Not!

Fasting is a very serious undertaking. Complete fasting with just water should only be done after some good research and the right mental, emotional, and intellectual preparation. That type of fast is not recommended for beginners.

The kind of fasting that I do has the purpose of cleansing. Lately, I have been having allergy symptoms with cough, post nasal drainage, and nasal congestion. It seems to be food related rather than environmental, so

I wanted to rest my immune system and digestive tract for one to four days. Then, I will slowly start adding food back into my diet to see if something is increasing the allergy load and causing the respiratory symptoms.

This kind of fasting is sometimes called a juice fast. Usually one would use vegetable juices. If you have a juicer, use carrot, celery, bok choy, spinach, and so on. Because I did not care to mess with the juicer, I used Green Zone by NSP, which is green vegetable powder. The drink consists of one liter of water, one scoop of Green Zone, one tbsp. flaxseed oil, one tbsp. honey, and 1/4 tsp. cayenne pepper. The Green Zone gives two to five servings worth of green vegetable fiber and nutrients. The flaxseed oil adds the necessary plant fats that provide some nutrient. The honey gives the mixture carbohydrates to prevent low blood sugar. And the cayenne helps the body stay warm. Drinking one liter of this mixture three times per day along with three liters of water provides a good cleansing of the digestive system and urinary tract while hydrating the body to release toxins that are trapped in the lymphatic fluids. Protein powder or amino acids can be added for nutrients.

For me, fasting also gives a chance to explore the feeling of hunger. Most of us never really have this feeling because we just keep feeding our faces at such a rapid rate that we never really experience hunger as a sensation in our body. Hunger is actually a healthy experience because it's designed to alert us to the fact that we need fuel. It does not mean immediately. Natural hunger is a good feeling, so we should not just jump up and get some food with every little twinge. When doing a fast, it is important to actually feel the hunger.

Most of the time when we get hungry, we begin converting stored glycogen and body fat into usable energy. Unfortunately, sometimes that system does not work and this conversion does not take place. When this happens, people begin to store food energy as fat instead of burning it. If there is no muscle added by doing exercises, then the body becomes more efficient because fat requires less maintenance energy than does muscle, and we begin to gain weight. Doing a fast can restart that normal conversion process.

For some people, doing a short fast of one or two days once per month is a good idea. However, you should check with your doctor before fasting, especially if you have any health issues. Begin by skipping one meal once in a while to see how that feels. Next, do a vegetable juice fast for one full day. Then try a little longer. At the beginning, I would suggest not fasting longer than four days. Do that a few times.

Also, read about fasting. Understand your purpose for doing this for your own health.

Doing cleansing meditations during this time has the added benefit of cleansing the mind as well as the body.

Eat Right for Your Type

The book *Eat Right for Your Type* by Dr. Peter D'Adamo was the first thing I wrote about when I started my newspaper column in 2006. Since then, we have seen a lot of very good results with the Blood Type diet.

Dr. D'Adamo's groundbreaking work with the connection of food and our blood type is somewhat controversial. The basic concept is that lectin, which is found in all food, combines with antigens, which are specific receptors on our red blood cells, to create either beneficial or harmful effects within our bodies.

These harmful effects come in the form of inflammation, joint and muscle pain, irritable bowel syndrome and gastro esophageal reflux disease (GERD), memory problems and depression, high cholesterol, and diabetes. The inflammation attacks our genetically weakest system. For example, the lectins in red meat are good for people with Type O blood, yet they cause inflammation in people with Type A blood. And A blood types need to eat lots of greens, fruit, chicken, and fish but not dairy, wheat, beef, venison, or pork. O blood types should avoid dairy, wheat, potatoes, and corn. B blood types should not eat chicken but usually can eat some dairy.

Wow, that sounds confusing. It is at first, but things do become clearer with practice. That also means that everyone is different, and all of the broad claims made by traditional medicine do not work for everyone. Most people with Type O blood should not be vegetarian, and the South Beach diet might work well for them.

We have been using this program since 2006. We have noted excellent results in control of weight, cholesterol, blood sugar, arthritis, and more.

Case Study: One man in his late 30s had cholesterol of over 300 and triglycerides over 3,000. After three months using the Eat Right for Your Blood Type diet, he lost 12 pounds and his cholesterol dropped to 230 with triglycerides at 350. This is still not perfect, but much better than before. Over the last two years, he has had ups and downs, but in general maintains nearly normal levels without taking medication.

Remember, as I wrote earlier in the section titled "High cholesterol is not a disease," these numbers for cholesterol are markers for inflammation, not the presence of a disease.

Read the book *Eat Right for Your Type* by Dr. Peter D'Adamo. Also his new book, *An Ounce of Prevention Is Worth a Pound of Cure*, in which Dr. D'Adamo gives more detail and a better understanding of why the Blood Type diet does not work for everyone.

Try this for yourself for four to eight weeks. Do not stop taking your medications. Just do this program 70 percent of the time. You will be amazed at how much better you feel and the improvement in your cholesterol and triglyceride numbers. As the results of your blood tests improve, then you can work with your doctor to reduce or get off your medication.

We should not diet to lose weight. Rather, we should learn to eat foods that benefit us and avoid those that harm us. When we do that, our bodies will become vibrant and healthy.

The Apo E Gene Diet

First discovered in the 1970s, the Apo E Gene has since been linked to conditions such as high cholesterol, heart disease, diabetes, Alzheimer's, Parkinson's, and multiple sclerosis (MS). Because the various Apo E genotypes affect how your body processes foods, eating a diet customized to your particular Apo E genotype will ultimately help reduce your risk of developing a disease associated with your genotype.

When you're eating for health, "one diet does not fit all," says Pamela McDonald, an integrative nurse practitioner and author of *The Apo E Gene Diet*. One reason for this is differences in the Apo E (Apolipoprotien E) Gene, which is responsible for determining how the body processes fat and cholesterol. In fact, the Apo E Gene diet is based on the concept that each of several genotypes process foods differently.

Genotypes

You inherit one of three naturally occurring gene variations, or genotypes, from each of your parents, giving you one of six possible pairings. Most people (64 percent) have the Apo E 3/3 genotype.

McDonald's own clinical experience, as well as mounting research, shows that among people who do not follow a healthy diet:

- *Apo E 2* is connected to high cholesterol, vascular disease, and Parkinson's.
- *Apo E 3* is linked to diabetes and insulin resistance.
- *Apo E 4* is related to inflammatory diseases like Alzheimer's and multiple sclerosis.

If you're interested in learning your genotype, you'll likely have to request a simple blood test or cheek swab through a private lab. Remember, carrying a particular disease-oriented gene does not mean you are guaranteed to get that disease. That's dependent on a whole host of factors, including lifestyles that influence your health. But by knowing your genotype and what conditions you are at risk for, you can help decrease these risks through tailored diet and lifestyle changes.

The Diets

Regardless of genotype, everybody benefits from eating an anti-inflammatory diet rich in antioxidants, healthy fats, fruits, vegetables, and whole grains. Another key is approaching food as fuel and eating small meals and snacks about every three hours. McDonald believes that determining the best "fuel" for your body depends on your genotype.

Apo E 2. For example, those with genotypes including Apo E 2 prefer fat and operate optimally with 30 to 35 percent of daily calories from healthy fats such as olive oil, avocados, nuts, and foods rich in omega-3 like salmon and walnuts. A sample dinner for this genotype carrier might be salmon, broccoli with chopped almonds, and a baked potato.

Apo E 3. This genotype processes fat normally and does best with a moderate fat diet, including slightly smaller portions of healthy fats, such as salmon, green beans, and brown rice.

Apo E 4. People with genotype pairings that contain Apo E 4 don't use fat for fuel very well and should aim for limiting it to 20 percent of total calories, deriving more calories from complex carbohydrates and plant proteins. Dinner could be beans, rice, avocado, and broccoli.

These might seem like small tweaks, but many of McDonald's patients have been successful, one even dropping 200 points from her cholesterol through diet and exercise alone. "This shows me that diet is so important that it should not be ignored," says McDonald.

She recommends making diet and lifestyle changes gradually to ease the transition and ensure they are sustainable. You will feel better and begin to lower your disease risk within just a few weeks.

For more information, visit www.thehealingcenteroflakeview.com or www.theperfectgenediet.com to find a practitioner who does this testing in your area.

Again, let your food be your medicine

The book by Dr. Bernard Jensen, DC, PhD, *Guide to Body Chemistry and Nutrition* repeats the advice of Hippocrates, the father of medicine. "Let your food be your medicine, and let your medicine be your food."

I know we have said this before, but we can't say it enough. If food selection, preparation, and cooking are done wisely, intentionally, and properly, very little time and money will need to be spent visiting health care facilities.

Knowing how to cook and what to eat plays a large part in our health and longevity. Innocent ignorance often leads to poor nutritional choices, deficiencies, and the kinds of diseases that prey on an undernourished body and shorten the life span. Heart disease, cancer, and diabetes all take a terrible toll on life in this country. All three are strongly influenced by food patterns and lifestyle habits. The right kind of knowledge can always lead us to a better life.

As health care providers, one of the hardest things to face is the resistance of patients who do not want to learn a healthier way to live. Many people want to have the doctor take care of them. They don't want to take responsibility for their own lives. We need to do more educating and less medicating, but that only works when people are motivated to learn how to take care of themselves. It is great to see the interest in this area begin to increase.

Nutrition doesn't stand all by itself as the path to good health. We need exercise, fresh air, water, spiritual time, sunshine, sleep, recreation, and time to stop and smell the roses. Drugs, herbs, acupuncture, homeopathy, surgery, chiropractic, and energy medicine cannot build new tissue; only proper nutrition can do that.

Learn how to select your food. Study food preparation and cooking so the healthier food will be tasty and appetizing. Taking time to sit down to eat with family and friends greatly enhances the body's ability to absorb and use the food. Remember, "Let your food be your medicine and let your medicine be your food."

Feed your body with proper nutrition

To work correctly, our bodies must have foods that contain all eleven primary chemical elements plus trace elements that are needed in tiny quantities. Soft tissues need oxygen, carbon, hydrogen, nitrogen, and sulfur. Boney tissues need calcium, phosphorus, and magnesium. The main electrolytes are potassium, sodium, and chloride. Essential trace elements include iron, fluorine, zinc, copper, iodine, selenium, manganese, molybdenum, chromium, and cobalt. Other trace elements that are not essential but very useful are silicon, vanadium, tin, nickel, arsenic, boron, strontium, lithium, and germanium.

Wow, that is quite a grocery list. All of that is supposed to come from our food. One of the big problems is that sometimes the soil in which food is grown does not contain all the things we need. For example, most Michigan soil is low in iodine. As a result, many people in the last few generations have had thyroid problems. This is why we feel quite strongly about supplementation of the diet with a good natural vitamin and trace mineral combination.

Another problem is picking fruit before it is ripe to increase the shelf life. I know someone who grows oranges, who picks them green and stores them for many months in cold warehouses. When it is time to ship them, the room is filled with some kind of gas that turns the peel from green to orange over-night. Sometimes, growers paint the oranges so they look nice. With such a masquerade, the fruit's nutritional content is difficult to know for sure.

This is why we strongly encourage you to buy organic if you can. Some of the local grocery stores are stocking organic foods; if they don't, ask and ask and ask until they do. Then buy them, of course.

Fruit and vegetables will have a sticker on them to indicate they are organic. On that sticker, look for a four-digit code that starts with a "9" (example 9253). This "9" means it is organic. 4000 numbers are not organic, and 8000 numbers mean the food is genetically modified (GMO). We do not really know yet if that is a big problem, but it might be.

The best advice is to eat organic and add a good natural vitamin plus a mineral supplement that includes trace minerals. We often add a cell salt combination, Bioplasma by Hylands. This contains all the ingredients needed to make structural elements in your body. Even though they are homeopathi-cally diluted but not succussed—that is, shaken like the homeopathic prepa-rations—they still absorb into the blood through the mouth. The twelve cell salts are: Calcium Fluoride, Calcium Phosphoricum, Calcium Sulphuricum, Kali (potassium) Muraticum (chloride), Kali Phosphoricum, Kali Sulph-uricum, Natrum (sodium) Phosphoricum, Natrum Sulphuricum, Natrum Muraticum, Ferrum (iron) Phosphoricum, Magnesium Phosphoricum, and Silicea (silica).

If you do take supplements, check to see if the tablet or capsule will dissolve in water or vinegar in less than five minutes. If it will, then it will dissolve in your digestive tract and be able to be absorbed. If it does not dissolve, you might want to use a similar supplement but from a different manufacturer.

Bone broth

When I was a young man, I remember watching my mother boil soup bones, ox tail, pig's feet, or chicken and turkey bones. I was just grossed out by this and the thought of eating food made in that way made me nauseated. So now, here it is many years later, and I am recommending bone broth for anyone with digestive disorders, especially irritable bowel syndrome, diar-rhea, colitis, Crohn's disease, and severe allergies. We have also seen great results with people who have emotional conditions like depression, anxiety, and bipolar disorder.

The concept of using bone broth for healing is very simple. It is a way to rest the gut or digestive tract for three to four days so it can heal. Once it is healed, the normal functions can return and eating patterns can be gradually advance back to normal.

The mental and emotional part of this is presented very well by Dr. Natasha Campbell-McBride, MD, who created the term Gut and Psychology Syndrome (GAPS). In her book *Gut and Psychology Syndrome: Natural Treatment for Autism, Dyspraxia, A.D.D., Dyslexia, A.D.H.D., Depression, Schizophrenia*, she shows how the digestive tract makes many of the neurotransmitters used by the nervous system. If the gut is not working correctly, those body chemicals will be out of balance.

Restoration of bowel function is essential for recovery of many normal body functions. Weston A. Price studied many primitive cultures who were extremely healthy. They all cooked and chewed bones, ground up bones and shells to powder, and added the powder to meals to get minerals and the structural elements to build healthy strong bones within their bodies.

So, how does one make bone broth? Very simple. Collect all your chicken or turkey bones. Put them in the freezer until you get enough to fill your slow cooker. You can also get them from your butcher by buying soup bones or oxtails. If you hunt, game animal's bones are very good. It is best if you can get your bones from personal sources, like someone who raises their own animals. This way there will be less toxins, antibiotics, steroids, and growth hormones in the bones. Cooking will destroy most of those toxins, but starting with good clean bones is better.

When you have enough bones, put them in your slow cooker. Depending on the size of your slow cooker, add enough water to cover the bones and one-half to one cup of apple cider vinegar (not distilled vinegar). Fill your slow cooker the rest of the way with healthy, non-chlorinated water. Then cook on low for 48 to 72 hours. Check and stir occasionally and add a little water if needed to keep the bones covered. After enough time, remove all the bones and discard them. Stir the broth. A lot of gel will float to the top. Do not discard this because your body will use that to build collagen or cartilage. Put the cooled broth in dated serving-size containers made of glass, ceramic, or hard plastic. Date the containers and put them in a freezer. If you need the broth now, use it. But make more as soon as possible so you have some available.

When using bone broth for cleansing, it is best to eat nothing but the bone broth and lots of water for two to three days. Warm the broth—but not in a microwave—and drink as much as you like throughout the treatment period.

After the two to four days, begin to add cooked veggies and fruit. You can drink the juices and water used to cook the vegetables.

Consume no raw vegetables or fruit for at least one or two weeks because raw fiber can be damaging to an irritated lining of the digestive tract. As you progress, you will feel better and then you can slowly begin to add raw fruit and vegetables.

Be sure to avoid all chemicals and additives.

Notice if any foods create problems when you add them back.

Good bugs and Candida

Many people do not know that our bodies are loaded with beneficial microorganisms, good bugs that help with our digestion and defense. These organisms are found in the digestive tract, the nose, mouth, sinuses, vagina, and skin.

One of the big health issues that face us today is the destruction of those good bugs. Antibiotics, chlorine in water, and antiseptic soaps are the major contributors to the losses of these friendly bacteria. When they are gone or reduced, problems can develop within our bodies.

Ask any woman who has had a yeast vaginal infection how she feels after taking antibiotics. Yeasts are often found in the vagina and in the digestive tract. They are dormant and held in balance by the good bugs. But when antibiotics kill the healthy normal bacteria, the yeasts have no competitors and grow wildly.

When this happens, many more problems occur. Most noticeable is the maddening itching of yeast vaginitis. But more detrimental are the toxins and waste products formed by these budding growing yeasts that cause irritable bowel syndrome (IBS) and interstitial cystitis (IC), chronic fatigue, allergies, fibromyalgia, headaches, memory changes, and much, much more.

Candida albicans is the name of the most common yeast found in our body. It is present in a dormant form in most of us, and it aids our digestion. But when it gets out of control, it causes many problems.

Unfortunately, it is almost totally ignored by the traditional medical community. I once went to an ears, nose, and throat (ENT) specialist for chronic sinus problems. He put a tube up my nose and into the sinus then sucked out some mucus. The culture showed a lot of yeast, Candida. He said not to worry because this was not significant, but it was very significant.

These yeasts clean up unabsorbed sugars in the last portion of the small intestine. If they get changed into their reproductive or budding form, they begin to produce toxic waste by-products that make changes in the cell membranes of our digestive tracts. This is called leaky gut syndrome, a condition that is not recognized by the traditional medical community.

When these changes in the lining of the digestive tract occur, we begin to reabsorb wastes that should be going down the toilet. Instead, they go back into the blood and need to be removed by the liver again. Because of the membrane changes in the small bowel, undigested proteins and sugars are absorbed into the blood. Our immune system recognizes these particles, which are too big to be utilized for energy, as foreign and begins to create antibodies against them. This leads to food sensitivity and our immune system to be either weakened or overly active.

The best way to keep the Candida yeast in dormancy is to eat a low-sugar/low-carbohydrate diet; add probiotics to your diet through organic, no-sugar-added yogurt, which is made with acidophilus, or other live probiotics; and avoid chlorinated water, pop, sugars, high-carbohydrate food, antiseptic soaps, hand gels, and oral antibiotics.

Calcium

As we get older, we need as much as 1500 to 2000 mg of extra calcium per day. The best food source of calcium is green vegetables; so eat lots of them.

There are two issues with lack of calcium. First, we need to get the calcium to absorb from the small bowel into the blood. Second, we need to transfer the calcium from the blood into the bones.

There are many different kinds of calcium. Each absorbs into the blood from the small bowel at a different rate.

Coral Calcium has the best absorption rate of around 90 percent, but it can make the body too alkaline and should not be used for a long period of time. Yet it might be good for people with Type O blood because they tend to be too acidic.

The most recommended calcium supplements are chelated calcium and calcium citrate. These absorb into the blood at an absorption rate of about 50 percent to 75 percent. I was taught that they are best if mixed with magnesium in a ratio of two parts calcium to one part magnesium, but the latest thinking is that a 1:1 ratio is probably better.

The worst absorption—and the cheapest, of course—is calcium carbonate and calcium lactate. Tums is made from calcium carbonate and is the product that many health care providers recommend to their patients for calcium supplementation. Yet only about three to ten percent of this calcium absorbs into the blood. Think about it: Tums was designed to neutralize stomach acid, and it must stay in the digestive tract in order to do that. But as long as Tums remains in the small bowel, it cannot be easily absorbed into the blood. So it's not really a good source of calcium for everyday needs.

People have been programmed to believe that milk is a relatively good source of calcium. Raw milk, straight from the cow, could be a calcium source, but it is illegal to buy raw milk in most states, and it is calcium lactate, which is not very absorbable. When I suggest that parents eliminate dairy from a child's diet, they always worry, "How will he get his calcium?" Then I ask them, "Where does a cow get its calcium?" From grass. So we should focus on greens as a source of calcium and leave the processed milk on the shelf.

The process of getting calcium from the blood into the bones is the next hurdle, and it is quite dependent on the pH level of the blood. The pH is a measure of acidity. The simplest way to measure this is to dip pH strips into saliva and urine every day for two weeks. The range of pH 6.5 to 7.5 is best for calcium absorption. Doing this can give you an indirect measurement of blood pH although it is not really very accurate. To avoid too much acidity, you must reduce red meat, tomatoes, oranges, pop, coffee, dairy products, and sugar.

By adding a cell salt supplement, Bioplasma, you can also enhance the absorption of calcium into the bones. Cell salts are in a chemical form that is easily absorbable into the blood through the mouth and then into the bone. Hormones do play an important role in absorption of calcium into the bones, but current thinking is that hormone replacement therapy (HRT) to improve bone density is too risky for the amount of benefit received. Bio-identical HRT is quite safe and can be used if needed.

Calcium is very important for many body functions, especially for bone structure. Get it from your food and greens then supplement with calcium citrate with magnesium if you need to. Be sure to balance calcium with magnesium. Calcium helps our muscles contract, whereas magnesium helps muscle relax. Heart arrhythmias, back pain, night leg cramps, restless legs often are relieved with magnesium supplementation.

Antioxidants: The fountain of youth?

Most people have heard of antioxidants. What is an antioxidant and why do we need them?

Any cell that uses oxygen for part of its energy gives off waste products. That is just like the engine in your car. Fuel plus oxygen creates energy and wastes. In the car, the wastes go out the exhaust system. Like your car, our body has a catalytic converter that also cleans up these waste by-products. The body uses antioxidants to convert these wastes into neutral compounds that cannot damage our body.

The wastes are often called free radicals. Mostly, these free radicals are created within our bodies, but some come in from polluted air, water, and food. Smoking, microwave cooking, and artificial preservatives create a lot of free radicals.

This is where antioxidants come in. They are molecules that have extra electrons to donate. They are like a car with two spare tires. When the free radical, which is like a car that's missing a tire, and the antioxidant meet, one donates and the other accepts and everyone is happy.

Usually we think of antioxidants as vitamin E, vitamin C, and those juice drinks like Xango, Thai Go, Noni, Ningxia Red, and others. These are, in fact, antioxidants and they do neutralize lots of free radicals. But most of the free radicals come from within our own cells, and these external antioxidants have very little effect on the internally generated free radicals.

Superoxide dismutase, better known as SOD, is an important antioxidant found in nearly all cells exposed to oxygen. SOD is an enzyme that converts free radicals to neutral, harmless molecules. SOD is generated in all cells that create energy from fuel and oxygen. So, the big question is, if SOD eliminates the free radicals made by our cells when energy is produced, then how can we get our body to make more of it?

Supplements of SOD have been around, but they are not very effective because they are proteins that get broken down in our digestive system. Again, these are too superficial.

More recently, intravenous (IV) glutathione has been shown to increase intracellular SOD, but that is very inconvenient and expensive, and many people just do not like the needles. Glutathione is an Nrf2 activator. Nrf2 is a protein molecule that enters the nucleus of a cell and turns on the process that makes SOD.

There are now some new NRF2 activator products that can be taken orally. They are a little pricey at around $50 a month, but a person could eliminate some of the other supplements and get a much better outcome. These products have been around for three or four years, and the results of research are looking very good.

My guess is that we are going to see great advances in this area of health care in the next few years. The product that looks best is Protandim. It is available through some health food stores and private distributors. The only side effect we have seen is dose-related diarrhea.

This probably is not the fountain of youth, but is it another way to put your health in your own hands.

Fats

To build healthy terrain and naturally protect ourselves from unhealthy microorganisms, we need good, healthy fats.

For the last 40 years, traditional medicine has been telling people to eat low-fat diets. As a result, everyone thinks that fats are bad.

Case Study: A few years ago, I saw a man in his 30s with erectile dysfunction. He told me he was on a very low-fat diet because his wife was also on a very low-fat diet and she did all the food preparation in their home. After checking his testosterone level and finding it to be very low, I suggested he put healthy fats back in his diet. In one month, all was working well again.

The truth is that fats are a very necessary part of our diet. The low fat trend has caused people to eat more carbohydrates, which have significantly contributed to the huge increases in diabetes.

We have all seen that ad on television that reminds us, "It is not nice to fool Mother Nature." I think we need to seriously follow that advice.

Cattle raised on grass, like nature intended, have very healthy fat with very little trans fats, while the fat in cattle raised in confined areas and on high carbohydrate diet is not. Fish that live in open waters have healthy fat—if not polluted with industrial chemicals like mercury and radioactive cesium-137—while fish raised on a fish farm have unhealthy fat with higher amounts of trans fats.

The real culprit is trans fats. What are those? The word trans refers to the shape of the fat molecule. The opposite shape is called a cis fat.

Trans fats are not normally found in nature and are difficult for the body to break down and utilize in healthy ways. They have been found to cause inflammation, which damages arteries, leading to plaque buildup and heart disease. Every cell membrane in our body is made up of lipoproteins, which are composed of proteins and fats. The fats should be in cis formation, which is what Mother Nature intended.

In general, trans fats were created and inserted into artificial cooking oils by the food industry in an attempt to improve shelf life in stores, make the oils into solids at room temperature, and thus reduce spoiling and those unpleasant odors that came from rancid butter. Crisco, released in 1911, was the first manufactured fat for cooking that contained partially hydrogenated oils and a high percentage of trans fats. Later, margarine came along and many other spreadable products that simulated natural butter followed.

Most doctors and scientists thought these products were safe and healthy. But it turns out that fats or butter from grass-fed cattle have a trans fat content of only two to four percent while Crisco, margarine, and buttery spreads have a trans fat content of 30 percent.

Our body can easily digest, burn, and utilize fats that come from Mother Nature. Olive oil, coconut oil, and flax seed oil are plant fats that are highly beneficial.

But even these, under high heat, become trans fats. So get rid of your deep fryer. Bake or broil your fatty foods. Use organic butter and stay away from all the artificial oils, butters, and spreads.

Fish oil and flaxseed oil are effective for reducing heart disease

The May 2008 issue of the Journal of the American Academy of Physician Assistants contained a good review article on the use of polyunsaturated fatty acids, also known as omega-3 oils as found in fish oil and flax seed oil, for prevention and treatment of heart disease.

The conclusion was that the use of oils containing omega-3 fatty acids:

- reduce the death rate in people with known heart disease
- reduce the number of abnormal heart rhythms
- lower total cholesterol
- reduce the death rate from all causes in the study group

Lowering fat in the diet actually had no impact on the death rate from heart disease. Whereas, in contrast, adding omega-3 fatty acids and 18 grams of fiber per day reduced death from heart disease by 29 percent within a two-year period. That is better than taking cholesterol-lowering statin medications.

I was quite impressed. This is the message that the natural health people have been promoting for many years.

Although not addressed in this research, there is some concern about heavy metal contamination of fish with mercury that are caught in the inland lakes and streams. Ocean mackerel, herring, and salmon caught in the wild have the highest levels of good fish oil per ounce of fish meat. Farm-raised fish have lower amounts of oil and a higher percentage of bad trans fats compared to wild-caught fish. Pacific Ocean fish may now have contamination with cesium-137 from the Fukushima nuclear plant leak of 2011.

In my opinion, it is actually better to use flaxseed oil than fish oil, mostly because of the contamination issue. Although the difference is subtle, it is significant because flaxseed oil contains more photon energy. Yet, some people think that fish oil or krill oil is better because of the type of essential fatty acids found there. Let me explain why I think the photo energy is better.

All our energy in the form of food comes directly or indirectly from the sun. Plant foods carry an energy vibration that matches the sun and is activated by the sun. Plant fats or oils are incorporated into every cell membrane of our body. Because these plant fats come directly from the sun and carry photon vibrational energy, they are activated when we get out into the sunshine or visualize sunlight or white light energy. This gives us direct energy from the sun. Fish oils are second generation and do not carry the photon energy. The science behind this concept is a little sketchy, but it comes from Dr. Johanna Budwig, PhD, who spent her life studying plant fats as a cancer treatment.

My own personal reason for liking flaxseed oil is because it does not seem to "burp up" as much as the fish oil. Both kinds of oil do have the beneficial effects as far as reduction of heart disease.

When you look at labels, look for abbreviations of the types of fatty acids that were found to be helpful: ALA, DHA, GLA, CLA, and EPA. This study recommends between 1000 and 4000 mg of these fatty acids per day in divided doses. Taking these with meals helps the digestion and absorption of these fats because bile salts and lipase are more available.

These good fats have been ignored because we have programmed people to think of all fats as bad and this is not true. It might be beneficial to have an Apo E Gene test done to see how much fat is ideal for your genotype.

Essential oils from seed to seal

In the summer of 2011, Barb and I had the opportunity to visit Young Living Farms in St. Maries, Idaho. This was a working vacation. On this farm of 200 acres, they grow lavender and melissa. These plants are harvested and the oil in them is distilled for use as essential oils. The melissa plants are cut using a swather and are loaded with pitchforks onto a large trailer. Then they are unloaded onto a large cement pad and allowed to "stress" for 12 hours. As the plants wilt, the availability of the oils increases. Then the plants are placed into a large steamer. The steam, which contains water vapor and oil vapor, is then cooled in a condenser. After the oil is separated from the water, it can be bottled and sold for medicinal use.

Because the melissa was not ready to harvest, we spent the first two days working in the green house, planting melissa seeds in small plastic seed trays. As these seeds germinate and grow into small plants, they will eventually be planted by hand in the fields where they can grow to maturity.

On the third and fourth day of our "vacation," Dr. Gary Young, ND, who owns the farm and is the founder of Young Living Essential Oils, decided that, because the melissa was not ready to be harvested, we would harvest balsam fir instead. This was done by going into a forest of balsam fir, cutting the trees and chipping them. The chips were then hauled to the distillery in a semi-trailer. The trailer was unloaded into a large steamer. The oil was steamed out of the woodchips, condensed, and separated from the water. We took the oil to the laboratory where it was stored and bottled. Half of a semi-trailer of wood chips made only about two gallons of oil.

The trees were cut using a large shear mounted on the front of the skid steer loader. They were carried to the chipper by another skid steer with the clam bucket. A small excavator was used to feed the trees into the chipper. The chipper, made by a Michigan company, Bandit Industries, blew the chips into the trailer.

The volunteers, like ourselves, were allowed to run all of these pieces of equipment. Most of the volunteers had never seen these kinds of machines, let alone operated them. So, for many, this was a peak experience, overcoming fear and reducing a large obstacle to something small and manageable.

Each night after working very hard in the fields and the woods, Dr. Young would spend a couple hours in the classroom relating his experience and knowledge about essential oils. We shared meals in a large comfortable lodge/mess hall and spent the nights sleeping in tents.

For the last 15 years, I've been using natural medicines, herbs, homeopathy, and occasionally essential oils. I never really understood that these oils are made by the plants to protect themselves from bugs, fungus, sunlight, and other natural dangers. This is why these oils have healing properties that we can use to improve our health. These properties include anti-inflammatory, anti-fungal, anti-bacterial, anti-viral, sedation or calming, energizing, and much, much more. So for me, seeing this process— from planting the seeds to sealing the oil in a bottle—was amazing.

On the last day of our vacation, Dr. Young and his staff took us up the St. Joseph River for an exhilarating white-water raft trip that ended with a nice barbecue. I am very grateful to Dr. Gary Young for providing this opportunity that any Young Living Essential Oil distributor can experience.

The Arthritis Cure

Many years ago, I read the book *The Arthritis Cure* by Dr. Joseph Theodosakis, MD. It was my first understanding that we can do something about joint pain besides taking Motrin and steroids. Since then, I have found many great ways to actually rebuild the joints.

This condition known as arthritis actually has a long period when people and their joints remain functional before actual pathology or damage to the joints occurs. But even the pathology can be reversed in many cases.

First, it's important to know that not all joint pain is arthritis, but that is the term we tend to call it. Actually, a joint has many parts and to fix the problem each part needs to be addressed.

The bone ends are covered with cartilage. This is covered with a slippery membrane called the synovium. Surrounding each joint are the capsule and ligaments that hold the bones in proper alignment. This lining of the joint capsule is filled with a lubricating gel made from hyaluronic acid. Running across the joints are tendons that connect the muscle to the bones. The bones are covered by a membrane called the periosteum to which the tendons attach. Inside the joints, underlying the tendons are bursa. These are small gel-filled sacs that act like pulleys to lubricate a variety of structures to make for smooth, pain-free operation. A problem with any of these tissues can cause pain in the joints.

The most common joint pains are caused by wear and tear of the cartilages, ligaments, and tendons that hold the joints together. It is important to note that all of these tissues are made of collagen, which tends to have very poor blood supply. As a result, most of the nutrients are diffused through the tissues and not through tiny capillaries like muscle, bone, skin, and so on. As a result, collagen structures tend to repair slowly. The slight concussion of mild exercise supports this diffusion of nutrients.

To make collagen, our body goes through many steps. Two of these steps produce chondroitin and glucosamine. If we add these directly to our diet, we can increase the production of collagen and repair our cartilages faster.

Dietary sources for chondroitin and glucosamine are the food product gelatin and animal cartilage or gristle from meat.

Most of us do not eat much Jell-O and most throw away the cartilage from meat. So adding a supplement that contains chondroitin and glucosamine will be very helpful. However, avoid chondroitin if you have a high PSA or prostate cancer. The third ingredient needed is methylsulfonylmethane (MSM), which helps break down the damaged collagen so it can be replaced with new.

All three of these supplements are in Osteo-Bi-Flex (OTC) or Ever Flex by NSP.

Another important nutrient is omega-3 from fish oil or flax seed oil. This acts as an anti-inflammatory and also helps in the production of the lubricating gel in the joint. Both fish oil and flaxseed oil have benefits, so we often recommend taking one or two of each once or twice daily. The production of lubricating gel can also be increased by dietary hyaluronic acid. We like Baxyl, the brand name for hyaluronan, which is a stable, absorbable form, unlike many other forms of hyaluronic acid

If you have spurs, which are calcifications of the ligament and tendon attachments, the joints will become stiff and painful, especially in the mornings. Small hard nodules often develop over the knuckles. These can be dissolved by using herbal Hydrangea three times per day and homeopathic Calcerea Carbonicum 6C or Hekla Lava 6C once per day. Depending on how many spurs are present, 80 percent of them can be completely dissolved in three to six months. Herbal treatments work best if you take an intermittent vacation from the herb. So we suggest taking Hydrangea only on days 1 through 25 each month.

Actions you can take to ease pain in your joints include:

- taking the supplements chondroitin, glucosamine, and MSM to repair the cartilage
- taking omega-3 oil and/or Baxyl to help your body make more lubricating gel
- taking hydrangea and homeopathic Calcerea Carbonicum 6C or Hekla Lava 6C to dissolve bone spurs
- following Dr. D'Adamo's Blood Type diet to remove inflammatory foods from your diet

- three to six months of exercising mildly with stretching and yoga, but no high impact exercise, which could cause more injury to the recovering joints

Fortunately, you do not have to take these supplements forever.

It is a good idea to take photos of your fingers before you start and then again later after they have improved. Send your pictures to The Healing Center so we can see the changes too.

Men's health

Many men have health issues they need to deal with. However, our culture has taught men that they have to be tough and not express any emotion. Many times, men are too embarrassed or afraid to bring up private health issues.

The introduction of Viagra as a pharmaceutical solution for erectile dysfunction has really been a great thing from the point of view of opening up some of the hidden issues of past generations. While I recommend many other alternatives to taking Viagra, this product and its advertising campaign has made men more aware of the health of their prostate. And that awareness is important because prostate problems will happen to all men at some time.

The prostate gland is like a donut. The urethra, which carries urine and seminal fluid, passes through the donut hole. The prostate grows until a boy reaches puberty and then it remains about the same size until age 50 or 60. Around that time, it gradually begins to grow again. The medical term for this is benign prostatic hypertrophy (BPH). As the prostate grows, the donut hole becomes smaller and urine stream decreases, making it more difficult to completely empty the bladder.

Erectile dysfunction (ED) has four causes: nerve damage, circulatory changes, hormone imbalances, and psychological worry about sexual performance.

Poor circulation is the biggest cause. Getting rid of stimulants, such as caffeine, pop, and tobacco, that cause constriction of blood vessels is the most important thing to do. Intravenous (IV) chelation therapy is often helpful to clean out toxins and blocked arteries. The Eat Right for Your Blood Type diet and the Apo E Gene diet helps reduce the inflammation in this area.

Spinal alignment by a chiropractor or massage therapist is generally beneficial to help the nerves work better. Using herbal Hydrangea and homeopathic Calcerea Carbonicum 6C to remove bone spurs can reduce spinal nerve problems associated with ED. Having a testosterone test done is beneficial to see if there are hormone deficiencies. Natural replacements are available if needed.

Several supplements are beneficial to help with ED: CoQ 10 improves circulation, X-Action for Men builds hormone levels, vitamin E (d-alpha tocopherol) increases circulation and decreases inflammation, L-Arginine increases nitric oxide, Suma helps all the endocrine glands stay in balance, and Zenn Plus is an herb combination that seems to work very well.

Having healthy bowel functions and open routes of elimination are very important to reduce toxins that might be affecting sexual function. Eliminating caffeine is absolutely essential for a healthy prostate. Saw palmetto is an herb that will shrink the prostate allowing the urine to flow better. Homeopathic Thuja 6C or Medorrhinum 12C has helpful residual effects for men who have had prostatitis and a history of sexually transmitted disease. Reducing the beer belly will reduce the level of estrogen, leading to a healthier prostate.

Case Study: HR came to The Healing Center with a complaint of frequent urination and a slow urine stream only at night. He did not want to take the prescription, Flomax, that his doctor had recommended. He had other issues that suggested food sensitivity such as post nasal drainage, chronic cough, and some heart burn at night. I suggested getting a food sensitivity test. Although a bit reluctant, he agreed to take the blood test for food sensitivity that evaluates 96 common foods. He reacted to 15 foods. To his delight, all of his allergy symptoms cleared by removing those foods from his daily diet. But, better yet, the urinary symptoms caused by an enlarged, inflamed prostate also got better. He was later able to determine that corn was causing the prostate swelling. And you guess it, he had been eating popcorn almost every night while watching television.

Remember to use proper diet and nutrition first, then try natural remedies, then supplements and then prescription medications to help maintain your healthy manhood. There are many things men can do to enhance sexual performance rather than taking Viagra.

Breast massage and testicular tapping

There are two things promoted by natural health practitioners and Chinese medicine that have proven to be very helpful for maintaining hormone health. The benefits have to do with balance and the increase of low hormones.

As we gracefully age, we begin to reduce the production of our hormones, which are estrogen and progesterone in women and testosterone in men. Women have premenstrual syndrome (PMS), early menopause, hot flashes, vaginal dryness, reduced libido, fat deposition on thighs and buttocks, loss of muscle mass, breast cysts, and other problems. Men have prostate problems that include cancer, erectile dysfunction, reduced libido, breast development, muscle loss, abdominal fat, among other issues.

The best natural method for reversing these things in women is breast massage and in men testicular tapping. These are very powerful prevention tools.

Women, once a day during your shower is a good time to perform this technique. Cup your breasts with your hands and move them vigorously up and down ten times, then side to side ten times, then around and around ten times, then around and around the other direction ten times. Using a rebounder or small trampoline or vibration plate, such as the commercial product Body Vibe, can also be very helpful to move sluggish lymphatic fluids from these tissues. See our site: www.thehealingcenteroflakeview.com for more information on the Body Vibe.

This exercise releases hormones from the hypothalamus, which is located in the brain, and will help rebalance all the female hormones. The other very important effect is to move the lymphatic fluid from the breasts, thus reducing the risk of fibrocystic breast disease and breast cancer. An important note here on a related subject, while the use of deodorants on the underarms is acceptable, don't use anti-perspirants because they plug up the sweat glands and might reduce lymphatic drainage from the breast, which increases cancer risks.

Men, during your shower, lightly tap one testicle with your finger tip ten times. Then do the other one ten times. Repeat this on each side for a total of 20 taps on each testicle. This increases male hormone production and has a balancing effect on the ratio of male and female hormones. Regular tapping reduces the risk of prostate cancer and enhances sexual performance.

I think you will find that these are important ways to prevent cancer in both men and women. And they are better than monthly examinations or periodic mammograms because the breast massage focuses on prevention while examinations are intended to detect cancer. In addition to that, the exercises balance the hormones to improve many aspects of life for both men and women. We have seen many cases of PMS completely go away with this technique, providing a great blessing for these women and their families.

Don't get me wrong, the breast exams should still be done. But ask yourself: Do you prefer prevention of cancer or detection of cancer? As I mentioned earlier in this book, what we focus on becomes our reality. So do you want prevention or detection?

When my articles about these wonderful prevention techniques appeared in the newspaper, some people were offended. Please know that my intention is to give people valuable tools to improve their health and their hormones without having to take medications and to promote the greater good of people in our communities.

I also recall as a child all the taboo and secrecy around these sexual issues. On one level, I understand that desire for privacy regarding certain parts of the human body. As parents, we want to protect our children from exposure to certain unseemly things, such as pornography, because the intention of those materials is usually disrespectful to the body and might be damaging toward relationships.

On the level of health and disease, however, all body parts have the same value. All parts of our body—even the parts that pertain to sexuality, propagation, and nurturing—need to be respected, maintained, and enhanced naturally. Prevention of disease in one body part is just as important as prevention of disease in another.

Influenza

With the outbreak of swine flu (H1N1) throughout the world in the spring and summer of 2009, we have become much more aware of influenza. Most experts agree that this was a pandemic, that is, a global event in which a virus can spread rapidly from person to person rather than an epidemic, which is a small, localized, expected event like the "normal" flu that comes every winter.

Fortunately, the swine fly was not very serious. As of August, 2009, there were about 40,000 cases in the US and about 300 deaths, mostly in the age range of 6 to 50. People over 60 were not targeted for the vaccine because most of them have some immunity from previous swine flu exposure. Less than one percent of the deaths were people over 60.

Swine flu and bird flu are so named because pigs and birds are the usual hosts for the influenza virus. The virus might spread to humans from these animals but usually not from human to human. When the viruses mutate, which enables them to spread from human to human, we then have the ingredients for a pandemic. You cannot get the flu from eating poultry or pork.

H1N1 influenza is caused by a virus. This virus is covered with spikes. One kind of spike acts like a hook, the first kind of spike is called a neuraminidase (the N in H1N1), which attaches the virus to a cell in the nose or lungs. The other kind of spike, hemagglutinin (the H in H1N1), pierces the cell membrane and injects its viral code into the cell. The cell's DNA is then used to make a more viral code, which is then used to make thousands of new viruses, which then are released to invade more cells and reproduce more viruses.

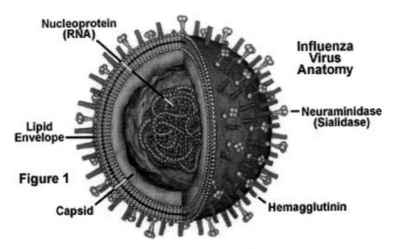

Figure 1

Nucleoprotein (RNA) · Influenza Virus Anatomy · Neuraminidase (Sialidase) · Lipid Envelope · Capsid · Hemagglutinin

The symptoms we experience come from our body's own immune system as it fights off the viral invasion.

- Mucus protects cells and prevents the virus from hooking up and penetrating the nose and lungs.
- Coughs and sneezes expel the virus from the body; coughing and sneezing also makes the viruses airborne and spreads them to others, so learn to cough and sneeze into your sleeve.
- High body temperature, or fever, kills the virus. Most viruses cannot live in an environment greater than 100.5 degrees, so do not treat a fever unless it is over 102. When ill, take hot baths to artificially raise the body temperature.
- Body aches keep us in bed, which is where we belong if we get this illness.

While good hand washing is important, these viruses are spread through the air, so the fanatical use of hand sanitizers is not necessary and might be detrimental because it kills the good bugs on our skin. Use plain soap and water. Gargle with warm salt water twice a day and use saline (salt) nasal spray two or three times per day. This helps break down the viral cell membranes if they are in your nose or mouth.

It is my hope that we never see a pandemic of some super flu. But I do hope people will educate themselves and perhaps be ready with some alternatives just in case there is a problem. There are several things that we can do to be ready.

Do not panic, just be prepared. Next we will share with you how to prepare, starting with a look at history. The Spanish Flu of 1918 was pandemic, an illness that killed an estimated 50 million to 100 million people around the world. There were units of the United States Army that were experiencing very high death rates from the flu. During that time in medical history, homeopathic medicines were quite popular and some Army units used homeopathy and herbs to treat the flu. These units had only a small percentage of deaths from influenza, whereas units that used aspirin and no homeopathy had death rates as high as 80 percent.

This tells us two very important things. First, if you get the flu, do not use aspirin, Motrin, and other non-steroidal anti-inflammatories (NSAIDS) to combat fever. There is some evidence from bodies frozen in Alaska from the 1918 Spanish Flu that a Reye's syndrome-like illness occurred with the flu and perhaps the aspirin caused many more problems than it solved. Reye's syndrome is a condition discovered in the 1950s. It was not until the 1970s that researchers determined that aspirin given to people with viral illnesses, especially children, developed a secondary illness that was almost always fatal. Tylenol (Acetaminophen) or homeopathic Belladonna 30C for adults or 30X for little kids and homeopathic Ferrum Phosphoricum 30C or 30X are much better and safer options to treat high fevers.

Second, have on hand some anti-viral, anti-flu herbal and homeopathic remedies. There will probably be a shortage when a pandemic comes, so it would wise to stock up now. It is not necessary to hoard large amounts of these medicines, just have enough for your family. They last for many years and are not expensive. Because of the way homeopathic medicines are prepared, a small quantity can be expanded into a large quantity of medicine very easily. Our website has a detailed explanation on how to do that: www. thehealingcenteroflakeview.com then click on bird flu/swine flu.

The two mainstay homeopathic remedies are Oscillococcinum and Gelsemium. In all, there are about 25 influenza remedies, depending on the symptoms, but these two are the main general remedies. Oscillococcinum is available in most health food stores and some pharmacies. If you cannot find it locally, you can get it from our website. It is more for prevention and is taken when flu is in your area. A box of Oscillococcinum, costing about $18, can protect a family of four people for 12 weeks. The usual dosage is one vial of granules once per week for prevention. To extend that, add one half vial of granules to four teaspoons of water, and then give one teaspoon to each family member once per week. Take the Gelsemium and other remedies after getting sick with the flu. These can be purchased at most health food stores or online.

Take lots of vitamin C, 500 mg three or four times per day. People with Type O blood should take vitamin C from rose hips; other blood types should take vitamin C from Acerola cherries. Cheap vitamin C, or ascorbic acid, has benefit but is usually hard on the digestive tract and often causes diarrhea.

Preventive remedies include herbs and essential oils. Taking echinacea and/or goldenseal at the onset of cold symptoms every day, days 1 through 25 of each month with five days off at the end of the month, seems to work quite well. Elderberry Defense, Immune Stimulator, and VSC, all by NSP, seem to help with viral infections in general. The essential oil, thieves, will kill the virus. Take this in lozenges, in tooth paste, direct application to a mask, or internally as two drops with two drops of olive oil in a gel capsule.

If you get the flu of any kind, H1N1 or seasonal, there is good treatment available using homeopathic medicines. Pick the one that best fits the symptoms.

- For body aches, fever, cough, runny nose, and headache, take Oscillococcinum 200 C, one dose three or four times per day until better, or for two or three days.
- For flu with fever, chills, body aches, dull feeling, droopy eyelids, and extreme weakness, take Gelsemium 200C one pellet twice per day for five days or 30C one pellet every two or three hours until better.
- For flu with vomiting, burning diarrhea, headache, restlessness and anxiety, take Arsenicum 30C.
- For slow onset of severe headache, irritability, and a desire to be left alone, take Bryonia 30C.
- For rapid onset of very high fever, headache, red face, and dilated pupils, take Belladonna 30C.
- For vomiting, take Ipecac 30C.
- For diarrhea, take Podophyllum 30C.

So do not be afraid, you can prevent and treat influenza without waiting for pharmaceuticals from the big boys.

Here it is again in outline form, this time with the remedy listed first. Photocopy this list and save it.

For prevention of influenza:

- Oscillococcinum, 1/2 vial once per week if flu is in your area
- Lots of vitamin C, 500 mg three or four times per day
- Echinacea/goldenseal days 1 through 25 of each month with five days off
- Elderberry Defense
- Immune Stimulator
- VSC, an herbal virus control formula made by NSP

- Essential thieves oil in lozenges, tooth paste, applied to a mask, or orally in capsules

For treatment, use these homeopathic products:

- Oscillococcinum 200 C, one dose three or four times per day until better, or two or three days
- Gelsemium 200C, twice per day for five days or 30C every two or three hours until better
- Arsenicum 30C for vomiting, diarrhea, headache, restlessness, and anxiety
- Bryonia 30C for slow onset of severe headache, irritability, and desire to be alone
- Belladonna 30C rapid onset of very high fever, red face, dilated pupils
- Ipecac 30C for vomiting and coughing until vomiting occurs
- Podophyllum 30C for diarrhea

Remember never use aspirin or products that contain aspirin when you think you have the flu. It might cause life-threatening Reye's syndrome in adults and children.

People often ask me what I think about flu shots. My approach is: Some people are highly sensitive and others are cast iron and never have adverse reactions. If you have been taking flu shots without any reactions, it is safe to continue. But if you have had flu shots and afterward experienced any flu-like symptoms like body aches, weakness, fever, and so on, then you might have increasing severity of reactions if you get more of them. That being said, you should re-read my comments in vaccinations and immunizations to look at the effects of the other ingredients in the vaccine.

Contact dermatitis from poison ivy

Once, a young man came to me with a case of poison ivy. This was in the early spring and the plants were still dormant, not even growing yet. Obviously, he was very sensitive. He had been working in the woods, wearing gloves and long-sleeve shirt. He got hot, shed his protective clothing, and came in contact with plants from last year that still carried the oil that causes the skin reaction.

The rash of poison ivy consists of blisters on a red base that are generally in lines. This is where the leaf rubbed across the skin leaving a trail of oil that then reacts with the skin in a sensitive person. The allergen in poison ivy is a substance called urushiol. In order to treat a reaction to the poison ivy, you need to neutralize the urushiol.

There are several herbs, when applied topically, that can do this. Jewelweed is one of the best. You can buy jewelweed soap. You can also combine this with any herb that contains a significant amount of saponins such as soapwort, horse chestnut, licorice, or rose leaves. Please remember that these are perfectly safe when used externally but saponins should not be taken internally, especially while pregnant or nursing. They are for topical use only. One thing to help control the itching is whole leaf aloe vera juice or gel. Cool baths with powdered colloidal oatmeal (Aveno) or Epsom salts can be extremely soothing.

There are several good homeopathic remedies that effectively treat contact dermatitis from poison ivy. Remember in all cases, the earlier the treatment the better. Homeopathic Rhus Toxidendron is made from poison oak leaves and will counteract the reaction to poison ivy. Homeopathic Croton Tiglium is a very good remedy for itching. Homeopathic Cantharis is good for any blisters, burns, or burning sensations.

The best treatment, however, is prevention. Avoid these plants. Here is what to look for: Three leaves. The center leaf is symmetrical with serrated edges. The two outside leaves are not symmetrical. The outside edge is serrated and the inside edge is smooth. Teach your children to recognize this leaf.

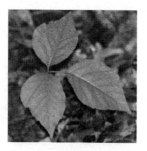

Poison Ivy

Wear long sleeves and gloves when working outside or walking in areas where you know or suspect there is poison ivy. After you are finished working outside, wash these clothes with hot water and detergent. The oil from poison ivy can get on tools, firewood, shoes, pets, and any inanimate object. Spraying objects with a soapy water solution will break up the oil and neutralize it.

Some people who have to work around these plants all the time will apply soap, like dish liquid, to their skin before going to work and rinse it off after work. This seems to break up the oil on contact with the skin. I am not sure how safe it is to have those chemicals on the skin all the time. Occasional use, I am sure, is fine.

Learn the plant, prevent exposure, treat naturally as soon as possible, and see your doctor if the natural measures fail.

Winter itch

By the time Christmas holidays come around, a lot of people are miserable with winter itch. This is a condition of dry, itchy skin, usually with some small red bumps and sometimes little pustules. Usually these are found on the upper arms, mid and upper back, chest and upper abdomen, and sometimes on the legs.

Most of the time, winter itch is related to a reduction of skin moisture and skin oil. It may also be aggravated by overheating parts of the body from heavy clothing.

The solutions are fairly simple.

- Run a humidifier in your home, especially in sleeping areas. Humidity should be between 45 and 65 percent. There should be a little condensation on the bottoms of the window panes, but not too much; that might ruin wooden window frames.
- Drink adequate chlorine-free water. Most adults should have between 40 to 60 ounces per day. Coffee, soda pop, and energy drinks are not water or adequate replacements for water. In fact, they are dehydrating and contribute to the problem.
- Reduce the temperature of the water in your bath or shower. Hot water removes some of the skin oils that are needed to lubricate the skin. Also, only soap and scrub the areas of your body that really

need to be scrubbed: feet, hair, armpits, bottom, and privates. Scrubbing the rest of the body removes much-needed skin oils.

- Add oil to your diet. For adults, two tablespoons of olive oil every day is helpful; these can be mixed in food. Omega-3 oil from fish or flaxseed, 2000 to 4000 mg per day with food in two or three doses, are highly beneficial for skin, hair, joints, and arteries.

In stubborn cases, vitamin E might be added. Natural vitamin E (d-alpha tocopherol), 400 IUs per day, is good. Be careful with synthetic vitamin E (l-alpha or dl-alpha tocopherol) because it could add to inflammation in your blood vessels. Over dosing vitamin E is not a good idea, so stay with 400 IUs of natural vitamin E per day.

Add vitamin A 25,000 IUs per day.

Finally, in states that don't get much winter sunshine, vitamin D3 is not necessarily needed to control the winter itch, but it is great for helping some other winter health problems we experience.

Toasted buns syndrome

Toasted buns syndrome is a condition of an itchy red rash that occurs on the low back, buttocks, and the backs of the upper thighs—thus its name.

It is a staph infection of the skin known also as folliculitis. This is caused by the heated seats in newer cars. The heat causes the pores around a hair follicle to open in an attempt to cool the skin. This allows normal skin bacteria and sometimes pathogens like methicillin-resistant staphylococcus aureus (MRSA) to get into the pore. When the skin cools after leaving the car, the pore closes, trapping the bacteria, which begins to multiply, causing a red and very itchy pustule.

Here is the solution. Turn the seat heater off after just a few minutes.

If you have this rash, take a warm bath daily with Epsom salts added to the water, and the rash will clear in four or days. Pretreat the Epsom salts with an essential oil blend like Purification, which has antibiotic properties.

Homeopathic first aid remedies for the summer

Many homeopathic remedies are made from herbs and plants. The dried plant is soaked in pure alcohol for a period of time and the resulting brew is called a tincture. To make homeopathic remedies, the tincture is then diluted and succussed (shaken) about 20 times with each dilution. If you look at the label of a homeopathic remedy, you will see "strengths" or potency, such as 6C or 12X, after the remedy name.

The 6 or the 12 represent the number of times the tincture has been diluted and succussed or shaken. The letter X indicates that the tincture has been diluted at a ratio of 1 to 10 (1:10). The letter C indicates that the tincture has been diluted at a ratio of 1 to 100 (1:100). The higher the number, the more dilutions, and the stronger it is. I know this does not make much sense, but in homeopathy, we are looking at the energy signature of the remedy not the physical substance from which the remedy is made.

Arnica Montana is a homeopathic remedy for sprains and strains. Most of the time, you will use a 30X or a 30C. This remedy is magic for any sprain or strain. This should be taken under the tongue every 30 minutes after the sprain, up to eight or ten times per day for an acute injury. If the injury is a few days old, use it three or four times per day. The recovery time is amazing.

Another great remedy for any household is homeopathic Apis 30X or 30C. This is made from ground-up honey bees. You guessed it, this works fantastic for bee stings. It is best to give every five to 15 minutes until the sting pain and swelling begin to subside. We have seen some great results with Apis on fresh and older stings with local allergic reactions.

If you have severe allergic bee sting reactions, get Apis 200C and an EpiPen, which is an epinephrine auto-injector, a medical device used to deliver a measured dose of epinephrine, most often for the treatment of severe allergic reactions called anaphylaxis. Keep these on hand and available. Immediately after a sting, take the Apis and head for the nearest emergency room, repeating the Apis 200C every five to 15 minutes.

Many times with the use of Apis 200C, the severe reaction will not occur and you will not have to visit the ER. Use the EpiPen only if you have trouble breathing or swallowing. If you do have to use an EpiPen, you must follow up in the ER because you will need further treatment.

Another excellent summer remedy is homeopathic Cantharis to treat sunburn and other thermal burns. Dissolve one or two pellets of homeopathic Cantharis 30C in the mouth every 30 to 60 minutes for acute sun or thermal burns. In addition to that, put ten drops of the essential oil Lavender into four ounces of whole leaf aloe vera juice. This can be applied topically with a little sprayer. Cantharis pellets, dissolved in the mouth, are also good for the burning feeling of a bladder infection.

For the weekend warriors with tendon strains, tendonitis, plantar fasciitis, and carpel tunnel syndrome, the remedy homeopathic Ruta Graveolans 30C, two or three times per day, has been very helpful.

Bug bites can be a big problem, especially for the little tykes. We use homeopathic Ledum 30X or 30C, one pellet before going outside or one pellet two or three times per day after being bitten. Ledum is also good for healing any puncture wound. (Remember, bites are punctures). The essential oil Purification is also very helpful to treat bug bites.

Spider bites will have a bruise around them and begin to ulcerate. The best treatment is the application of heat as hot as you can stand to denature the protein in the venom. But be careful not to use so much heat that you burn the skin.

So enjoy a safe spring and summer, but if you do have some mishap, it is better to be prepared. We suggest a general remedy kit. These are available at most health stores and carry about 20 of the most commonly used homeopathic remedies for acute situations.

Case Study: A few years ago, Barb and I were on vacation. My cell phone rang, and on the line was a frantic grandmother who was watching her granddaughter have a fever seizure. I knew she had a remedy kit. I asked if she had homeopathic Belladonna. Yes, she did! She placed the quick-dissolving tablet inside the child's cheek. In less than 30 seconds, the seizure stopped. Within 15 minutes, the fever was gone. And the child was up and playing in less than an hour. They did not even have to go to the ER. Preparation and some education about these remedies is a great thing.

A basic remedy kit might contain the following: Aconite, Apis, Antimonium Tartaricum., Argentum Nitricum, Arnica, Arsenicum Album, Belladonna, Bryonia, Calcerea Carbonicum, Calendula, Cantharis, Carbo Vegetabilis, Chamomilla, China, Drosera, Gelsemium, Hepar Sulphuricum, Hypericum, Ignatia, Ipecacuanha, Kali Bichromicum, Lachesis, Ledum, Lycopodium, Magnesium, Phosphoricum, Mercurius, Natrum Muraticum,

Nux Vomica, Phosphorus, Pulsatilla, Rhus Toxidendron, Ruta, Sepia, Silica, Staphysagria, Sulphur.

An explanation of uses of all of these is beyond the scope of this book. A good homeopathy book for beginners is *Homeopathic Remedies for Health Professionals and Laypeople* by Blair Lewis, PA-C.

Arnica: Homeopathic wonder drug

This remedy should be in every home in the 30C or 30X potency. It is made from the herb leopard's bane, also known as mountain daisy, which grows in mountainous areas. The whole plant, including the roots, is ground up and soaked in alcohol to make a mother tincture.

The tincture is poisonous and should not be taken orally, but it can be used topically for injuries. The homeopathic form is very safe and is made from the tincture by diluting and shaking the desired amount of times. 30C potency is diluted 1:100, 30 times. The 30X potency is diluted 1:10, 30 times. Between each dilution it is succussed (shaken) approximately 20 times.

This remedy is fabulous for treatment of sprains, strains, contusions, bruises, and any kind of musculoskeletal injury because it speeds up the natural healing mechanisms. Ankle sprains that would normally take four to six weeks to heal will be better in one or two weeks.

It is also used to reduce pain and complications during and after surgery. Take one pellet under the tongue the night before surgery, one the morning of surgery, and one four to six times per day after the surgery, depending on the amount of pain. The results are remarkable. Countless numbers of our patients use this and have no need for pain medications after surgery.

Most surgeons are unaware of these products and do not want patients to use them, so you probably will have a little resistance. Coach your doctor ahead of time so there are no problems.

Case Study: GVB had a diseased gallbladder and needed surgery. She took one homeopathic Arnica 30C the night before surgery, one pellet the morning of the surgery, one when the hospital staff took her to the operating room. After recovery, she had no pain at all and had to take only one additional pellet.

258 Put Your Health in Your Own Hands

This remedy is also really important for head injuries. Any head injury, no matter how mild, should be treated with homeopathic Arnica. The effects of mild to severe head injuries can be cumulative and can be responsible for symptoms like memory changes, loss of sense of direction, and loss of concentration. All of these will improve with use of this wonder drug after head injury, even if the head injury occurred long ago.

Using this will allow the internal healing mechanism to help the brain to fully recover from the injury, leaving no residual to accumulate with the next whack on the head. Try it and you will be amazed.

Remember, you can also use homeopathic Naturum Sulphuricum 30C once per day for a month or so to help with resolution of old head injuries.

Tonics

When I was a young boy, I remember my mother giving us a tonic called tiger's milk, which tasted awful. I have no idea what was in that drink. Now, as I study more natural health, I am beginning to hear about the use of tonics to improve the terrain so the body can function normally and restore health naturally. And I'm beginning to suspect that Mom was on to something that she knew was good for me.

Below are seven signs of health:

1. Clarity: to have understanding and clear thinking
2. Adaptability: to take whatever comes, like with martial arts to easily evade or catch spears being thrown at you
3. Well-being: to have a generally healthy feeling without the need for artificial stimulants such as a cigarette or a cup of coffee
4. Calmness: to go with the flow and handle stressful events with competence
5. Strength: to be physically strong and emotionally stable
6. Energy or vitality: to feel full of energy and confidence
7. Order: to have inner peacefulness and a neat personal space

If you have most or all of these signs of health, you are on the correct path. If you have only one or two of these signs, perhaps you need some help.

Changing some habits would be beneficial and using a tonic or two can be very helpful.

A tonic is defined as:

- An agent, such as a medication, that restores or increases body tone
- An invigorating, refreshing, or restorative agent or influence
- A substance that stimulates physical, mental, or emotional vigor

Below are examples of a few tonics that have proven to be highly beneficial on people's journeys back to great health.

1. *Morning Green Drink:* Drink this first thing in the morning
   4 to 8 oz. water (may be warm or cold)
   1 capsule probiotic
   1 scoop Green Zone or any green drink supplement
   2 tbsp. organic lemon juice or ¼ fresh squeezed lemon or lime
   ¼ to ½ tsp. of baking soda (do not use baking powder)

2. *Bedtime Tonic:* Drink 15 to 30 minutes prior to bedtime
   4 oz. warm almond milk or hot water
   1 to 2 tsp. black strap molasses
   ¼ to ½ teaspoon baking soda or one tablet of Alka-Seltzer Gold
   (not regular Alka-Seltzer because you do not want aspirin or
   acetaminophen in this tonic)

3. *Apple Cider Vinegar* for pH balancing
   1 or 2 tbsp. between meals once or twice per day
   Or 1 tbsp. at beginning of meal to assist with digestion of protein

4. *Oil Pulling* for detoxification
   Before brushing teeth or drinking water (perhaps while showering): Swish 1 or 2 tbsp. of Sesame or Sunflower Oil in your
   mouth for 10 to 20 minutes, then spit it out.

5. *Maple Syrup and Baking Soda,* a cancer treatment support tonic
   Mix 1 cup 100 percent pure maple syrup and 1/8 cup baking

soda in a small sauce pan and heat for five minutes. Take 1 or
2 tsp. of this mixture daily.

6. *Flaxseed Oil and Yogurt*, the Budwig Cancer Support Tonic
   Thoroughly mix 4 tbsp. liquid flaxseed oil with 1 cup yogurt or
   organic cottage cheese. Eat ¼ of this mixture 1 to 4 times per
   day depending on your state of health.

7. *Chia Seed Gel* for nutrition and appetite control between meals
   Mix 1 part chia seeds in 9 parts water and 1 part organic juice
   for flavor.
   Take ¼ to ½ cup of the resulting gel between meals twice a day.

8. *Hydrogen Peroxide* to reduce inflammation
   Dilute 3 percent hydrogen peroxide in an equal part water. Place
   this mixture in a small spritzer bottle and spray 5 sprays in
   your mouth 4 to 5 times per day

9. *Ningxia Red with Essential Oils*, an antioxidant
   1 to 2 oz. Ningxia Red made by Young Living Essential Oils.
   Add Young Living Essential Oils for specific treatment.
   Drink once per day at bedtime.

Use your intuition or muscle testing to determine which of these tonics
alone or in combination with others will help you find your way to perfect
health. Each of these has a specific function, which I will explore next.

Morning Green Drink
   4 to 8 oz. water (may be warm or cold)
   1 capsule probiotic
   1 scoop Green Zone or any green drink supplement
   2 tbsp. organic lemon juice or ¼ fresh squeezed lemon or lime
   ¼ to ½ tsp. of baking soda (do not use baking powder)

Many people do not eat breakfast. That is what I used to do. No breakfast. Just grab a Diet Coke, a king size Baby Ruth, which I justified by saying

that I was getting protein from the peanuts—what baloney!—and finish that off with a big chew of Red Man tobacco. All while driving to work. I was fatigued all day and had to keep ramping up the energy with coffee, Coke, sweets, and tobacco all day long. Then at night, I was so over-amped, I could not sleep.

Most of us do not eat enough green vegetables. Who has the time to buy, clean, prepare and eat five, that is right, five servings of green vegetables every day? That is what we need to offset the acidic foods and junk we eat every day. Even if you have a great healthy salad for lunch, it is not enough.

There are many green drinks available. Most of them give the equivalent of five to seven servings of vegetables. A little lemon gives the liver a jump start, the baking soda balances more acidity, and the probiotic puts good bacteria back into the digestive tract. Some people add a raw egg, protein powder, or chia seeds. You can have it your way. Be creative. It might take a few weeks to readjust your body chemistry, but you will begin to feel true vitality.

Bedtime Tonic

> 4 oz. warm almond milk or hot water
> 1 to 2 tsp. black strap molasses
> ¼ to ½ teaspoon baking soda or one tablet of Alka-Seltzer Gold (not regular Alka-Seltzer because you do not want aspirin or acetaminophen in this tonic)

This is an interesting beverage that is used often in the south. I listed it as a bedtime tonic, but many people use it as a mid-morning pick-me-up as well as an evening drink. When used with almond milk, it has a taste similar to cappuccino, but is much healthier at a fraction of the cost.

Start with the warm almond milk or hot water.

Add the molasses next. Molasses is the refining by-product of making sugar. It is loaded with calcium and iron but only has five grams of sugar per teaspoon. And it is much more alkaline than coffee. It has no stimulant effect like coffee other than the comforting heat associated with drinking a hot beverage.

Next add the baking soda. This further alkalizes the drink. Much of our daily food intake of meat, dairy, citrus, tomatoes, potatoes, yeast foods, sugars, and so on are very acidic. The baking soda is used to offset that, reducing inflammation. Baking soda adds a bit of bitterness to the drink. So, if you like strong coffee, add a little more baking soda to mimic the taste of coffee. ¼ to ½ teaspoon seems to be both beneficial and tasty. Be careful not to use baking powder. The effects will not be desirable.

Some people add Alka-Seltzer Gold. This product is hard to find, but you can get it over the internet at www.drugstore.com. Regular Alka-Seltzer has aspirin in it, so avoid that and use Alka-Seltzer Gold. This gives a little fizz to the drink, but I found it to be too bitter for my taste.

Remember the idea of a tonic is to provide an invigorating, refreshing, or restorative influence. This tonic does that, and it has some of the comfort qualities of drinking a cup of coffee without the risk. So experiment with this. You just might make a new friend.

Apple Cider Vinegar

> 1 or 2 tbsp. between meals once or twice per day
> Or 1 tbsp. at beginning of meal to assist with digestion of protein

Apple cider vinegar is a great tonic for improving health. It is an effective, natural, bacteria-fighting agent that contains many vital minerals and trace elements such as potassium, calcium, magnesium, phosphorous, sodium, sulfur, copper, iron, silicon, and fluorine that are vital for a healthy body.

Natural apple cider vinegar is made by crushing fresh, organically grown apples and allowing them to mature in wooden barrels. This boosts the natural fermentation qualities of the crushed apples, which differs from the refined and distilled vinegars found in supermarkets. When the natural vinegar is mature, it contains dark, cloudy, web-like sediment called mother that becomes visible when the rich brownish liquid is held to the light. Natural vinegars that contain this mother have enzymes and minerals that distilled vinegars from grocery stores do not have due to over-processing, over-heating, and filtration.

For this reason, it is recommended that you purchase only natural apple cider vinegar, which has an ideal acidity (pH) level of 5 to 7.

Natural apple cider vinegar is a wonderful natural remedy for a number of ailments that usually require antibiotics and other medications that have a number of side effects. One teaspoon of apple cider vinegar, when taken on an empty stomach one or two times per day, has been known to:

- Reduce sinus infections and sore throats
- Balance "bad" and "healthy" cholesterol
- Help with skin conditions such as acne
- Protect against food poisoning
- Aid digestion of proteins
- Fight allergies in both humans and animals
- Prevent muscle fatigue after exercise
- Strengthen the immune system
- Increase stamina
- Increase metabolism that promotes weight loss
- Alleviate symptoms of arthritis and gout
- Prevent kidney and bladder stones and urinary tract infections

When taken, one teaspoon at the beginning of a meal, apple cider vinegar can improve digestion and reduce constipation. This is especially true for people who do not have enough hydrochloric acid in their stomach to convert pepsinogen to pepsin to break down proteins. If you take one teaspoon at the beginning of the meal and it increases heartburn and reflux, do not continue to take the apple cider vinegar before meals. In this case, a little bit (1/4 to ½ tsp.) of baking soda in two ounces of water will usually fix the heartburn with meals and not interfere with the digestion process. Too much baking soda will cause rebound heartburn. That means it will initially improve, but when it comes back, it will be much worse than before.

Oil Pulling

Before brushing teeth or drinking water (perhaps while showering): Swish 1 or 2 tbsp. of Sesame or Sunflower Oil in your mouth for 10 to 20 minutes, then spit it out.

Oil pulling or oil swishing, in alternative medicine, is a traditional East Indian folk remedy that involves swishing oil in the mouth for oral and systemic health benefits.

The ancient Indian yogis used oil or their own saliva, swishing it around in their mouths as part of a spiritual healing ritual. More scientifically, it has been shown that oil pulling is able to remove fat-soluble toxins, particularly hydrocarbons, like herbicides and pesticides, from the blood vessels in the floor of the mouth. The exact process of this is not really well understood, but it seems that oil or fat-based toxins have been found in the oily foam after the procedure is completed.

The procedure is this: In the morning before brushing your teeth, swish and rinse your mouth with approximately one tablespoon of oil (sesame, walnut, or sunflower oils are the most recommended) for ten to 20 minutes. Then spit it out. Do this first thing in the morning before eating or drinking so that your stomach is empty.

At first, I only used one teaspoon. I started with five minutes while I was taking my shower or shaving. Now I use more oil and do it easily for ten or 15 minutes. At first, I gagged on the oil but not anymore. I spit the oily residue into the toilet because I wasn't sure how the trap in the sink's plumbing would handle the oil.

This swishing process helps the oil thoroughly mix with saliva. As you continue, the oil gets thinner and white. The oil is put in the mouth, with chin tilted up, and slowly swished, sucked, chomped, and pulled through the teeth. The oil changes from yellow and an oily consistency to a thin, white foam. If the oil is still yellow, it has not been pulled long enough. After spitting the oily foam from your mouth, rinse your mouth with water, spit that out, and then brush your teeth normally. This procedure is best performed once every day.

Another benefit is that this tonic exercises the facial muscles, which helps with muscle tension headaches, pain in the jaw joint, and might reduce facial wrinkles. There are reports of improvement in teeth and gums, but I have personally not seen that yet.

If you have had exposure to toxic chemicals, facial muscle problems, history of stroke or Bell's palsy, or mouth problems, I think this tonic would be quite helpful. Some people say it is helpful for chronic fatigue and fibromyalgia. I am not really sure about that, but it is certainly worth a try for a few months.

Maple Syrup and Baking Soda

Mix 1 cup 100 percent pure maple syrup and 1/8 cup baking soda in a small sauce pan and heat for five minutes. Take 1 or 2 tsp. of this mixture daily.

This is one of those tonics that has emerged from folk medicine in the hills of East Tennessee and North Carolina. In that area, folk healer Jim Kelmun, also known as "Dr. Jim," has been recommending this for many years. Dr. Jim discovered this treatment accidentally somewhere in the middle of the last century when he was treating a family plagued by breast cancer. There were five sisters in the family and four of them had died of breast cancer. He asked the remaining sister if there was anything different about her diet, and she told him that she was partial to sipping maple syrup and baking soda.

Since then, as reported by a newspaper in Asheville, N.C., Dr. Jim has dispensed this remedy to more than 200 people diagnosed with terminal cancer. Amazingly, he claims, of that number, 185 lived at least 15 more years and nearly half enjoyed a complete remission of their disease.

Traditional medicine would argue that something so simple could not possibly work. But the mechanism of action is very interesting. When mixed and heated, the maple syrup and baking soda bind together. The maple syrup targets cancer cells because they consume 15 times more glucose than normal cells. The baking soda, which is dragged into the cancer cell by the maple syrup, is very alkaline. This forces a rapid shift in pH or acidity, thereby killing the cancerous cell.

Dr. Tullio Simoncini, an oncologist from Rome, Italy, acknowledges that cancer cells gobble up sugar. So when you use this tonic, it is like sending a Trojan horse into your cellular structure. The sugar is not going to encourage the further growth of the cancer clusters because the baking soda is going to kill the cells before they have a chance to grow.

Some of you might have heard of PET scans, which is a short name for positron emission tomography. These scans are used for progress studies for prognosis in cancer patients. Radioactive tracers are attached to glucose and then given to the patient in an IV solution. Because cancer cells love sugar, the tracer soon is taken up by the cancer cells and it can be detected on the PET scan.

This principle suggests two things: first, the maple syrup/baking soda tonic has a scientific basis; and, second, diets that contain a high sugar and high starch content are likely to feed cancer cells. So cut the carbohydrates and take a teaspoon of the tonic every day. It can be preventive or therapeutic. It cannot hurt and it certainly could help.

Flaxseed Oil and Yogurt

> Thoroughly mix 4 tbsp. liquid flaxseed oil with 1 cup yogurt or organic cottage cheese. Eat ¼ of this mixture 1 to 4 times per day depending on your state of health.

For over 40 years, a German doctor, Johanna Budwig, PhD, has been studying the effects of diet and sunlight for the treatment of cancer. She has been nominated six times for the Nobel Prize in Medicine.

We typically think of cancer as strong and overwhelming. But Dr. Budwig's work shows that cancer cells are really weak and cannot survive well in the presence of oxygen. This has been confirmed by numerous other studies. So, if we can oxygenate the cancerous tissues, they will die.

Dr. Budwig found a way to increase the oxygen in all cells. The basic formula is very simple. All of our body's cell membranes are made up of lipoproteins, which are a combination of fats and proteins. The quality of the fats that make up these lipoproteins determines how much oxygen can be transported into the cell through the cell membrane. If these fats come from trans fats or saturated fats, they cannot transport oxygen very well. Cells need cis fats, or highly unsaturated fats, and the best sources of these are seed oils like flax seed oil.

These oils, unfortunately, are very unstable and become rancid very easily. If you grind flax seed, it must be used within one hour. If there are any liver or gallbladder issues, it is hard to get these good oils absorbed and into the cell membrane where they can transport oxygen.

Dr. Budwig discovered that mixing the flaxseed oil with the protein from low-fat cottage cheese or yogurt, before eating it, solved both problems. The protein will bind with the flaxseed oil to make a stable, water-soluble lipoprotein that does not become rancid quickly and is easily absorbed and assimilated into the cell membrane. Because it is no longer a fat, it can be absorbed directly rather than having to be processed with bile salts.

Using this daily will greatly increase your body's cellular oxygenation, and cancer cells will not be as able to survive. For prevention, use one tablespoon of good flaxseed oil in one quarter cup of organic low-fat cottage cheese or yogurt once per day. Fresh fruit or organic honey can be added for taste. For treatment, make up four tablespoons of flax seed oil per one or two cups of cottage cheese or yogurt and eat some of that four times per day.

To ensure a good mix, it is best to use a blender rather than simply stirring. In addition to this tonic, it is essential to avoid *all* trans fats. Deep fried foods are a major source of the bad trans fat. So go easy on the fish and chips. If you do eat those deep fried foods occasionally, use a fat grabber with that meal.

Fat grabbers are herbal combinations that bind fats so they cannot be absorbed into the blood. Use with caution because they can cause diarrhea that looks like the grease from taco meat. Eat grass-fed beef and free range chicken if you can. They have less than five percent trans fat in the meat, compared to 40 percent in factory farm or feedlot livestock.

Google the Budwig Cancer Diet for many references and more details on this program.

Chia Seed Gel

Mix 1 part chia seeds in 9 parts water and 1 part organic juice for flavor.

Take ¼ to ½ cup of the resulting gel between meals twice a day.

Most of us have heard of Chia Pets. But there is something much more important about the chia seeds than being used to make the Chia Pets.

In 2009, an amazing book, *Born to Run* by Christopher McDougall, came on the scene. The subtitle of this book tells it all: *A Hidden Tribe, Super Athletes, and the Greatest Race the World Has Never Seen.* The Tarahumara tribe from Copper Canyon in northern Mexico is a relatively hidden group of cliff dwellers who run everywhere they go. As part of their tradition, they run races—not 26-mile marathons, but 100 and 500 mile races. They often run bare foot or in sandals made from old rubber tires. The shoe giant Nike tried to get some of them to wear running shoes. Most of the shoes only lasted about ten miles, being kicked off and replaced by their sandals.

The most interesting thing about all of this is what they eat when they are running these long races. You guessed it: chia seeds and water. For our purposes, we suggest you add the chia seeds to water and let them stand for ten to 15 minutes. The covering softens and the fiber inside unfurls, releasing a gel. This gel is loaded with nutrition—proteins, good fats, and very little carbohydrate. This can be mixed with yogurt or fruit juice. Or drink it as is.

On the website, www.getchia.com, William Anderson wrote a very nice article called, "Chia Seed, the Ancient Food of the Future."

Dr. Mehmet Oz, MD, has become a national spokesman for those exploring many natural and alternative health-related products. He says, "The truth is, Chia seeds are actually good for you—we're talking really good for you! In fact, they just may be one of the healthiest things around. Here's why: Nutty-tasting whole-grain Chia seeds are loaded with omega-3 fatty acids, and they have among the highest antioxidant activity of any whole food—even more than fresh blueberries. And they do good stuff for the body, like keeping blood pressure and blood sugar under control."

Nutrition expert Dr. Andrew Weil, MD, says: "I enjoy the seeds' nutlike flavor and consider them to be a healthful and interesting addition to my diet. You can sprinkle ground or whole chia seeds on cereal, yogurt, or salads; eat a handful of whole seeds as a snack; or grind them up and mix with flour when making muffins or other baked goods. You can make your own drink, called a Chia Fresca, which is popular in Mexico and Central America: Stir 2 teaspoons of the seeds into 8 to 10 ounces of water (you'll end up with a slightly gelatinous liquid). Add lime or lemon juice, sweeten with xylitol or stevia to taste, and enjoy."

The bottom line is that chia seeds are highly beneficial and will make a great nutritional addition to your daily diet. If stored in a cool dry place, they last forever.

Hydrogen Peroxide

> Dilute 3 percent hydrogen peroxide in an equal part water. Place this mixture in a small spritzer bottle and spray 5 sprays in your mouth 4 to 5 times per day.

There have been many articles written about using peroxide to oxygenate the body and thus improve health. Lots of people in the natural health movement use Food Grade 35% Peroxide mixed with another liquid in what is known as "drop doses" and claim amazing benefits. The chemical formula for water is H_2O and peroxide is H_2O_2. When peroxide splits, it leaves oxygen and water, both generally safe and beneficial substances. That is what causes the bubbling action of the peroxide.

Dr. Grant Born, DO, from the Born Clinic in Grand Rapids, Michigan, always told me to be very careful because too much oral or intravenous peroxide could cause oxidation (instead of oxygenation), which causes a lot of inflammation and damage to our blood vessel walls. As a result of those conversations, I have always stayed away from the use of peroxide even though it is reported to be highly beneficial. The difficulty was controlling the amount of peroxide so there was no damage and only benefit.

A few years ago, we were introduced to a technique that seems to remove my concerns about the over-dosage of peroxide. Regular strength, three percent peroxide is diluted with equal parts water or a natural mouth wash and sprayed into the mouth. This will safely improve the oxygenation of the blood by absorbing some of the oxygen from the peroxide through the mucous membranes of the mouth. It is important to know that this does not improve oxygen in the blood in the same way the lungs do. It will also act as an antiseptic to help eliminate viral and bacterial infections.

This is also helpful for people with cryptic tonsils who accumulate little curds of food and debris in those pockets in the tonsil. Spraying and gargling will get the peroxide into the crypt and the bubbling action will loosen the curds. Regular use of this technique for three or four months will shrink those large tonsils.

Dr. Robin Murphy, ND, my homeopathic mentor, states that he has seen great results with this simple little tonic. I have been using this daily four or five times per day for about six months. It appears to be safe and very beneficial for prevention and treatment of chronic diseases and maybe some cancers.

Ningxia Red with Essential Oils

1 to 2 oz. Ningxia Red made by Young Living Essential Oils.
Add Young Living Essential Oils for specific treatment.
Drink once per day at bedtime.

This is the tonic Barb and I use every night for our "bedtime toddy." We use chilled Ningxia Red, an antioxidant drink made by Young Living. You can use any of the other antioxidant drinks that are popular like Xango, Thai Go, Noni, but we prefer Ningxia Red.

Any pure essential oil can be added to the drink as a way to take them orally. Make sure your oils are pure and can be safely used internally. Some essential oils are made by extraction, using solvents like hexane to separate the oil from the plant or from the floral water, which is a by-product of the steam distillation process. In that process, some of the solvent, hexane, remains in the oil. These solvents are harmful hydrocarbons that can be neurotoxic. Also some essential oils are cut with castor oil and other oils to extend them. So beware and only use pure essential oils. Do not believe the label until you have researched the manufacturing process.

Barb and I use essential oils like Thieves, which is anti-fungal, anti-viral, and anti-bacterial, and Digize, which breaks down hydrocarbons, pesticides, and herbicides. We often use others oils in the tonic, depending on our needs for the day.

This tonic has a great taste and is physically and mentally a great way to enter our night rest and rejuvenation period of the day. It is much healthier than an alcoholic nightcap.

You can order these products directly by going to: www.thehealingcenteroflakeview.com, clicking on products, and then clicking Young Living Essential Oils.

Conclusion:
Put Your Health in Your Own Hands

A S we come to the conclusion of this book, I want to leave with you some of my final thoughts about maintaining a positive attitude and outlook as you apply the practical information I've presented so far.

You are so lucky!

As Barb and I were getting ready to leave on a vacation to Hawaii, many times, I heard these words. "You are so lucky. We can't afford to do that." The truth is, I am lucky, but not in the sense that most people mean it. My definition of luck is: "Priorities and Planning Meet Preparedness." We decided about two years earlier that we wanted to take a trip to Hawaii because neither of us had been there before. We set that as our priority. And we began to plan! We saved money. We watched for deals on airfare and accommodations.

So think about this process. You make a decision to do something. In your mind, you see yourself there and you automatically begin the creative process. If you never decide to go, nothing will ever happen. So, the first step is the choice to do it.

The next step is to ask: how much moolah are you going to need to make this happen. This is preparedness.

Money is also called currency. Like a current in a stream, it implies flow and movement. Money is a renewable resource. In order for money to do something for you, it must move and go somewhere or to someone in exchange for what you desire. Currency does you—nor anyone else—any good in your pocket. But to take a trip, you need to accumulate some *deniro* to exchange for that trip. You do not want to do this on a credit card. Save up front, so the entire trip is all paid for when you go. The memories are then not clouded by the stress of paying the credit card bill.

Let's say you need $5,000. For most of us, we look at that and feel overwhelmed. We often think, "I just do not have that kind of money. You are lucky to be able to afford that, but I cannot afford it." So look at your budget. Ask yourself, "How can I afford this?" Where could you squeeze out a few bucks each month to begin accumulating some *jing* for that trip?

Here are a few places in our daily lives where we could make some changes. Some people smoke. At, let's say, $5.00 per pack, which is $150 per month or $1,800 per year. If you go out for dinner to even a modest restaurant or to the movies once a week for $30, you are paying out $1,500 per year.

I used to party once a month or more and spend easily $50 each time, so that is $600. Most people spend $50 to $150 per month on cable television. If you cancel that service and turn off the tube, at the average rate, you have another $1,200 per year. How many of us buy doodads all time, junk that we do not need? Many of us spend $2 to $5 per day for coffee and snacks. That's another $1,000 per year you can save by packing a lunch instead of eating out. Ka-ching. Once you look, there are lots of possibilities.

So, you have the three Ps: Priority, Planning, and Preparedness.

Once you decide to go on your trip, to recharge your solar batteries and see the world, you must make some priority decisions to budget the flow of your currency into the trip fund—or whatever special fund you choose. It might take two or three years to build up your "fun" fund, but it will be well worth it.

When you begin thinking like this, things happen. Barb and I found a great deal on a cruise that was half the usual price. That happened because we were prepared, not because we were lucky. You can experience something like that too—if you're "lucky" in the "priority, planning, preparedness" sense of the word.

Changing your thinking like this is also great for your health. You eliminate a bunch of really bad, unhealthy habits and convert them into life-changing, mind-expanding experiences.

The law of the garbage truck

A few years ago, Barb and I took a trip to northern Michigan and I picked up a local newspaper from one of the small towns along the way. In it was this article and I am passing it along. The author was not identified:

One day I hopped into a taxi and we took off for the airport. We were driving in the right hand lane when suddenly a black car jumped out of a parking space right in front of us. My cab driver slammed on his brakes, skidded, and missed the other car by just inches.

The driver of the other car whipped his head around and started yelling at us.

My taxi driver just smiled and waved at the guy. I asked, "Why did you do that? This guy almost ruined your car and sent us to the hospital. Why were you so friendly?" This is when the cab driver taught me the "law of the garbage truck."

He explained that many people are like garbage trucks. They run around full of garbage, full of frustration, full of anger, and full of disappointment. As the garbage builds up, they need a place to dump it and sometimes they will dump it on you. Don't take it personally. Just smile, wave, wish them well, and move on. Don't take their garbage and spread it to other people at work, at home, or on the streets. Don't even mention it.

The bottom line is that successful people do not let the garbage trucks take over their day. Life is too short to wake up in the morning with regrets. I used to love to tell my sad story for the day: the flat tire, the speeding ticket, the slip and fall. But now I realize that I was just seeking attention. It did nobody any good to pass on the sad story of the day. So stop doing that, especially on Facebook.

Love the people who treat you right and pray for the ones who don't. Life is ten percent what you make it and ninety percent how you take it. Have a blessed, garbage-free day.

And thank you, to that unknown cab driver for the lesson that how we think and what we think about has a huge impact on our health.

Happiness

What is happiness? The Bill of Rights of the US Constitution guarantees the right to pursue happiness. It does not guarantee happiness, just the pursuit of happiness. But many of us have found that the pursuit of happiness is not a very happy experience. We often are conditioned by our culture, parents, and the media by images of what happiness should look like. We see television commercials for everything from prescription drugs to sporting events to a new car, all promising to make us happy.

If we look at happiness from a body chemistry point of view, it is a flood of chemicals, manufactured by several organs in the body, that creates a feeling that we have labeled "happiness." This chemical process is very complex and it includes hormones and neurotransmitters like adrenaline, serotonins, and endorphins. In spite of the amazingly complicated chemistry involved, we can create this feeling by having a thought that moves a few muscles in our face into a smile. Yes, all we have to do is smile, and our body knows how to do the rest.

People who know me know that I often whistle. I usually do not even know what I am whistling. Sometimes, it is a Christmas tune in July. Years ago, someone asked me, "Why do you whistle all the time?" My immediate response was, "Because I am happy." But after giving this some thought, I realized that the opposite is true: I am happy because I whistle.

Wow! What an insight. This means that I can change my body chemistry simply by whistling. And so it is. We can create happiness by smiling, singing, whistling, humming, and all sorts of other triggers. We do not need outside help. We can create happiness within ourselves by simply thinking happiness and smiling. We do not need the latest new car, dream home, island vacation, cruise, prescription drug, alcohol, or that fabulous pair of shoes to be happy. Happiness is internal, not external.

The permanent feeling of happiness is related to a sense of satisfaction. This is a sense of comfort and wellbeing. This is a knowing that everything will be alright. Things are okay. All is well.

Many of us have worries about the future. Living in the future causes only fear and frustration. Living in the past might create anger and bitterness. Be thankful for everything that has happened in the past because that is what brought you to this point and it is all good. Living in the past or the future sucks the joy right out of us.

The best way to create happiness and satisfaction is to spend a little time in the future, planning and imagining the way you desire things to be. Remember the past only to recall the lessons you learned, and then return to the present and live life with a sense of wonder and gratitude. I know a young man who recently lost his job. At first, he was angry and resentful. However, he soon made a shift. He understood that every ending is also a new beginning. It is an opportunity to start something new and be happier than before. Not surprisingly, within weeks he found employment that was better than his former job.

We hold the secret. Happiness is a choice. Make it happen right now. Smile. Laugh out loud. Enjoy life, moment by moment right now.

The attitude of gratitude

The following is an article I wrote the week before Thanksgiving Day, 2012, entitled "The Attitude of Gratitude."

Thanksgiving Day is a day set aside to be thankful for our blessings. According to history, this was started by early settlers in Massachusetts to celebrate a great harvest and blessings in spite of the hardships of coming to the New World. Today, this holiday is full of football games and over-eating. I think we should go back to the original intent of this holiday. I think we should stop and think for a few minutes about being thankful for many great people and things in our lives.

All of the great religions teach gratitude as an important part of our spiritual welfare. Being grateful to God is of highest importance. Being thankful also has mental and emotional benefits. Our self-esteem and self-worth are extremely important for sound health. How we feel about others is reflected in how we feel about ourselves. When we have good self-esteem, we will naturally see more worth in other people and we will be more grateful to others, just for being themselves or for what they do for us.

It is important that we appreciate our family, even though we might not like some of them and we might get into a fight over Thanksgiving dinner. That relative who we do not care for is here to teach us some kind of lesson. As soon as we turn our focus from what we do not like to what we would really, really like, we will move away from negative feelings about that person and become nicer. Perhaps they will be nicer too and maybe they will just move to a different city. What really happens is that we change and they simply follow our lead.

We must be thankful for our work. Work is an amazingly beneficial activity. It also increases our self-worth because we can look back, see, and feel good about what we have accomplished for the day. We must be thankful for the men and women who produce the businesses that provide everything we use in our daily lives. These producers provide services and jobs so we can eat and care for ourselves and our children. These business people are grateful for the consumers who buy their goods and services. For the unemployed, Thanksgiving, as well as every day out of a job, is a difficult time. But these people, and all of us, can be grateful for assistance from others in our community and in our churches.

Last week, a man came into my office and was complaining that the President was a socialist. I laughed out loud because I knew this man was on Social Security disability, Medicare, and Medicaid. His defensive reply was that he had been injured and "could not help it if he could not work." After a brief discussion, he understood that he should be thankful for the social programs and "socialist" Presidents who started these social welfare programs for people who temporarily need help. In spite of lots of complaining about our government and the country, we still live in the best nation in the world. Be thankful you live in America.

It really does not matter what our situation is, we can be grateful about many things. We just need to look at our life and our situation in a different way. I would like to challenge you to stop for a few minutes and think of at least 20 things for which you are thankful. Include people in your life. Write them down and tape your list to your calendar for the current month; if it is near the end of the month, then tape your list to the next month also. Periodically look at your list and express your gratitude for each and every person or item there. Then, at the end of the next 30 or so days, sit down with your list and make another list of events that have happened in regard to the items on your initial list. You will see that many good things have happened in those areas of gratitude. That's because when you focus on a thankful feeling, you will attract to yourself more things for which you can be grateful.

The Attitude of Gratitude is a powerful tool that will help us spiritually, mentally, emotionally, and financially.

The Art of Being

I recently read *The Art of Being* by Dennis Merritt Jones, DD. He has a companion eBook, *Seven Be-Attitudes*. I would recommend reading both of these. With his permission, I am sharing a synopsis of the seven Be-Attitudes below.

1. **Be Present in Every Moment.** You are invited to "be" rather than to "do."
2. **Be Willing to Listen to your Intuitive Self and the Guidance it Offers.** The primary difference between the animals and us is that they cannot choose to ignore that guidance, but we can and often do ignore it. When we ignore it, we often suffer the consequences of that choice. Hearing and listening are two different functions.
3. **Be Open and Transparent in your Communications.** Transparency means you have nothing to hide, nothing to defend, and nothing to fear.
4. **Be of Service to Others.** A life of wholeness will never be obtained until you offer the whole of yourself to the whole of life.
5. **Be Generous and Grateful.** Someone who has developed the attitude of gratitude and generosity is first and foremost established in an attitude of "I am enough." There is an inherent intelligence in nature that knows there is always enough for everyone.
6. **Be Reverent.** We begin to awaken to the idea that there is really no place where God's presence begins and ends.
7. **Be Unconditionally Loving.** Unconditional means there are no conditions attached. It is tempting to draw circles around certain people that are more "lovable and deserving" of our love than others. Focus on what someone is, not on what they are doing.

How we think about others and how we think about ourselves has a huge impact on our physical health. Being some or all of these seven Be-Attitudes will greatly improve the quality and quantity of your life. His summary of this concept is that these are "Seven Ways of *Being* that Will Alter the Altitude of Your Attitude." [Emphasis added.]

I am thankful to Dennis Merritt Jones for his amazing insights.

Dennis Merritt Jones produces a great monthly newsletter. To receive the newsletter, go to www.dennismerrittjones.com.

You can be, do, and have anything you desire

Many years ago, I was given a copy of a book *Think and Grow Rich* by Napoleon Hill. This book was a turning point in my life. It was the first time I understood that my thinking could make a difference. Up until then, I thought I just had to accept what happened and react as best I could. But this book said I could cause things to happen if I thought about them in a particular way. It was exciting because I found that it worked. Finances, health, relationships, and career opportunities were affected by my thoughts.

Later, I heard the statement, "One could be, do, or have anything that he or she desired." I sort of glossed that over, thinking, "Yeah. Yeah. I know all that stuff." Well, that statement turns out to be so true and so powerful that it is hard to believe. And I really did not understand it at all at that time.

So let's take a minute to break this down.

We *have* things and possessions that cost money. We also *have* relationships that do not cost money but are very valuable. And we *have* family; these are people we don't own, but they are our family whether we like them or not.

How did we acquire any of these things? By *doing* something. Nothing happens until we do something, putting forth action of some sort: working, talking, selling, driving, studying, reading, listening to speakers, going to college, taking training courses, cooking, cleaning, building, waiting, serving others, writing, loving, and so on. When we do something, the results are having something: possessions, relationships, cars, homes, toys, friends, family, a bigger bank account. Successful actions result in having those things that we desire.

How do we know what successful action to do in order to acquire the things that we desire? Somehow, we have to learn that.

Earlier in this book, I wrote two sections titled "You are what you eat" and "You eat what you are." The concept is that we act, based on "who we are." Here is an example, let's say two people witness someone stumble over a curb and fall on the sidewalk. One of the witnesses is an emergency medical technician (EMT) and the other one is an accountant. Because of who he is, the EMT knows exactly what to do. The accountant probably does not know what to do. So their action is based on who they are.

Who we *are* is based on all of our past experiences, good or bad. We are a cumulative composite of everything we have ever experienced. It is important to understand that we can change who we are. We can eliminate the effects of traumatic events of our past. We can enhance the things that have been good. We can begin to listen to people who do and have what we desire or who have been where we are now and grown beyond that point. We can educate ourselves. We can get a mentor who can teach us to *be* and *do* so that we can *have* the things and types of relationships we desire.

This process of be, do, have is very simple and sequential.

First, we become the person who we desire to *be*. Those traits will then cause us to *do* the actions that will attract things into our life that we desire to *have*. If we try to force the actions before we become that person, we will fail because our thoughts and actions will be incongruent and will not have any attractive power. If we possess things without becoming that person or doing correct actions, we will be very unhappy, living outside of our comfort zone, and we will sabotage everything until we lose those things we had.

Remember you can be, do, or have anything you desire. It is up to *YOU* to learn how.

Healing and health care

Many years ago, Dr. Bruce Bennett told me, "In the field of medicine, there are healers and there are technicians; you must learn to be both." At the time, I was not sure what he meant, but over the years his words proved to be a great bit of insight. I have continued to study and learn in both of these areas.

Technology is the area of medicine that traditional health care has been following. Surgery, pharmacology, laboratory tests, and medical imaging have advanced tremendously in the last 30 years, and costs of care have skyrocketed along with that. (Isn't it interesting that the cost of an MRI in the US is $1,700 to $2,000 compared to $160 in Brazil?) But in spite of the negatives, I am still amazed every day at the lifesaving procedures that the technology of medicine can perform.

I do not always agree with the way prescription medicines are used in this country. The drug industry has had a huge influence on the education of health care providers, and many times, medical practitioners are coached by them to try to micromanage body chemistry to create a specific outcome. In some cases, that coaching and the prescribed pharmaceuticals are necessary. But I think the traditional medical community has lost sight of the fact that the body can heal itself in most cases, and they have simply accepted unwanted side effects as part of the benefit of the drug.

Natural health practitioners have seen huge advancements in the technology also. There are thousands of new computers, sensors, and treatment devices. Technology has also helped us gain more knowledge about and produce more effective herbs and supplements. At the same time, there has been a resurrection of many of the old and ancient methods that still have validity. With the increased understanding of quantum physics, we are now better able to understand what is happening with energy medicine.

In homeopathy, for example, the energy signature from a plant is captured by a remedy preparation and now is able to be transferred to a person or pet to heal symptoms that match the remedy. There is no simple explanation at the present time for how and why this works, but I am sure it is related to quantum physics.

At first, it was difficult to overcome logic and make the leap of faith necessary to use things when we did not know how they work. On the other hand, traditional medicine does not really know exactly how most prescription medicines work either. So maybe faith in the unknown is not too much of a stretch after all.

I used to watch Dr. Bennett just sit at the bedside of a very ill patient, sometimes all night, and many times the patient would get better even though the good doctor really did not do anything, or seem to do anything. He never could explain it, but he would just say, "Sometimes the patient just needed someone there."

That seemed very strange to me as a new physician assistant graduate, who had been taught in school that I and my colleagues were to heal the world with drugs and surgery. Now I understand that Dr. Bennett was, in some unknown way, truly a healer in addition to being a good technician. He was one person who had a great positive influence on my life and my career. Through his eyes, I saw now how we can have so much success with homeopathy.

Holistic medicine at The Healing Center of Lakeview

Holistic medicine (I wish the word was spelled "wholestic") is a system that looks at the *whole* person and incorporates all the aspects of traditional, natural, and homeopathic medicine, depending on what the person needs. Dr. Bruce Bennett once told me, "Use everything available. If a person has back pain, send them to a chiropractor first, not a surgeon. But if the patient has appendicitis, send them to the surgeon, not the massage therapist."

So it is with "wholistic health." And so it is at The Healing Center. We use many different modalities to help people achieve and maintain good health, according to their individual needs at that time, as they strive for perfect health.

I am a certified physician assistant, trained in traditional medicine. But for 20 years, I have been practicing natural health. Barb, my wife and business partner, is a certified massage therapist and natural health consultant with 15 years of experience. We are both certified natural health practitioners (CNHP), which means we can provide traditional and natural health assessments. We also both work with energy medicine using Reiki, hands-on healing, emotional releasing, and more. I do hypnosis and genetic memory healing. We both have extensive training in counseling and guidance.

We know and use tried-and-true methods, but we also believe in not simply doing the same old thing over and over again year after year. No, we have been training and educating ourselves, constantly upgrading and improving our skills, keeping pace with ongoing advancements in natural health care.

We use homeopathy, Bach Flower remedies, and naturopathic medicine techniques, which include nutrition, supplements, and herbs. We make recommendations for prescription medicine, surgery, nutrition, vitamins, minerals, supplements, cleanses, herbs, massage, hypnotherapy, dream work, chiropractic, homeopathic remedies, and energy work.

My book and audio CDs are designed to work with the mind-body-spirit connection. By using these, our patients can learn to relax and manage stress, augment cancer treatment, eliminate undesirable habits, and help their children to concentrate and focus.

Put Your Health in Your Own Hands

You now have completed the journey that I spoke of at the beginning of this book. So let's look back and see what we remember and what we have learned.

Putting your health in your own hands is the "wholistic" concept we must embrace as the world shifts in consciousness. We are learning to gather ourselves together, to muster all of our parts: body, mind, emotions, and spirit.

It is my intention that you use this book as a reference to become responsible for your own body. To do that, I have introduced you to the following ideas that we must expand and study if we are to have long, healthy, productive lives:

- Cleanse our bodies of toxins
- Stop adding to the toxic load
- Rebuild the damaged tissues
- Control our minds
- Learn to focus and concentrate
- Slow down and relax our minds
- Enhance our memories
- Use our negative emotions to focus on what we really, really want
- Feel good all the time
- Connect with our spirit, with the spirits of other beings on this earth, and with the spirit of our Higher Power

This book is a tool, a starting place, a beginning. My purpose is to introduce you to the possibilities and help you step a little bit out of the box; to awaken your consciousness a little bit more to understand your full potential;

to give you one more little nudge toward self-awareness and understanding that you have unlimited potential; to know that you can be, do, and have anything you desire to be, do, or have.

All you need to do is put your health—physical, mental, emotional, and spiritual—in your own hands and then muster all your parts into an integrated whole.

PUT YOUR HEALTH IN YOUR OWN HANDS!

Appendix

Contact information and website links

The Healing Center of Lakeview
332 S. Lincoln Ave.
Lakeview, Michigan 48850
(989) 352-6500 (O) (989) 352-6273 (F)
www.thehealingcenteroflakeview.com
bobhuttinga@healingcenter.biz

Alka-Seltzer Gold for use in tonic: Google www.drugstore.com/alkaseltzer-gold

Apo E Gene diet, information and testing: www.theperfectgenediet.com

Bach Flower Remedies: www.thehealingcenteroflakeview.com, click Products, then Bach Flower Remedies

Bio-identical hormone replacement: www.thehealingcenteroflakeview.com, click Services, then Bio-Identical Hormone Replacement

Body Vibe, whole body vibration plate: www.thehealingcenteroflakeview.com, click Products, then Body Vibe

Chia seeds to purchase: www.getchia.com

Cholesterol and the use of statin medications: http://diabetesupdate.blogspot.com/2008/11/should-you-be-taking-statin-what.html

Dennis Merritt Jones newsletter: www.dennismerrittjones.com

Dr. Bessheen Baker, Naturopathic Institute of Therapies & Education: naturopathicinstitute.info

Dr. Joseph Mercola's newsletter: www.mercola.com

Dr. Sherri Tenpenny's vaccine information: www.drtenpenny.com

Dr. John Lee, Bio-identical hormone replacement therapy: : www.drjohnleemd.com

Food sensitivity testing: www.thehealingcenteroflakeview.com, click Services, then Food Sensitivity Testing

Glycemic index from Harvard Medical School: http://www.health.harvard.edu/newsweek/Glycemic_index_and_glycemic_load_for_100_foods.html

Homeopathy, 12 homeopathic remedies to know: www.thehealingcenteroflakeview.com, click Products, then Homeopathy

Homeopathy, Find a homeopath near you: www.nationalcenterforhomeopathy.org

Influenza: www.thehealingcenteroflakeview.com, click Bob's Blog, then Bird Flu, Swine Flu

Milk, Campaign for Real Milk, a project of the Weston A. Price Foundation: www.realmilk.com

Mind Coaching CDs: www.thehealingcenteroflakeview.com, click Products, then Mind Coaching CDs

Nature's Sunshine Products: www.thehealingcenteroflakeview.com, click Products, then Nature's Sunshine Products

Tapping techniques EFT and TFT, as described by Dr. Gary Laundre: http://www.thehappinesscode.com/12345.pdf

Vertigo: www.youtube.com, search for Epley Maneuver

Young Living Essential Oils: www.thehealingcenteroflakeview.com, click Products, then Young Living Essential Oils

Virtual Gastric Band Hypnosis, find a practitioner: www.sheilagranger.com

Weston A. Price Foundation: www.westonaprice.org

Index